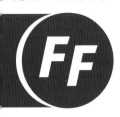

*AST FACTS*

**FF**

*dispensable*
*uides to*
*linical*
*ractice*

# Low Back Pain

### Robert L Swezey

Director, The Swezey Institute
Santa Monica, California
and Clinical Professor of Medicine
University of California at Los Angeles
USA

### Andrei Calin

Consultant Rheumatologist
Royal National Hospital
for Rheumatic Diseases
Bath, UK

HEALTH PRESS

Oxford

Fast Facts – Low Back Pain
First published July 2003

Text © 2003 Robert L Swezey, Andrei Calin

© 2003 in this edition Health Press Limited
Elizabeth House, Queen Street, Abingdon, Oxford OX14 3JR, UK
Tel: +44 (0)1235 523233  Fax: +44 (0)1235 523238

Book orders can be placed by telephone or via the website.
For regional distributors or to order via the website, please go to:
www.fastfacts.com
For telephone orders, please call 01752 202301 (UK) or
1 800 538 1287 (North America, toll free).

Fast Facts is a trademark of Health Press Limited.

A CIP catalogue record for this title is available from the British Library.

ISBN 1-903734-34-7

Swezey, RL (Robert)
Fast Facts – Low Back Pain/
Robert L Swezey, Andrei Calin

Medical illustrations by Dee McLean, London, UK.
Typesetting and page layout by Zed, Oxford, UK.
Printed by Fine Print (Services) Ltd, Oxford, UK.

Printed with vegetable inks on fully biodegradable and
recyclable paper manufactured from sustainable forests.

444    001

Low emissions
during production

Low
chlorine

Sustainable
forests

# Glossary

**Allopathic:** This term is used here to describe conventional diagnostic and therapeutic procedures, but was originally taken from the term 'allopathy', which is based on homeopathic theory that by producing symptoms of a second condition presumed to be antagonistic to the first, a positive therapeutic outcome can be achieved

**α-receptors:** Large nerve fibers in the peripheral nervous system that serve as mechanoreceptors to stimulate proprioception and also pain

**αβ-receptors:** Somewhat smaller fibers than α-receptors that, like them, are mechanoreceptors and transmit proprioception and vibration

**Bone morphogenetic protein (BMP):** A substance that is injected percutaneously into a bony structure and in particular into the vertebral body to stimulate bone formation and fracture repair

**Bursa:** A closed envelope-like sac lined with synovial membrane containing a thin layer of fluid. These are found in regions subject to friction, such as a bony prominence where a tendon passes over the bone

*Ischial gluteal bursa* lies beneath the gluteus maximus muscle and the inferior aspect of the ischium

*Subgluteus maximus trochanteric bursa* lies just beneath the gluteus maximus muscle over the inferior slope of the greater trochanter

**Bursitis:** Inflammation of a bursa

**Cauda equina:** A bundle of nerves descending vertically from the lumbar, sacral and coccygeal spinal nerves which somewhat resembles the tail (cauda) of a horse (equina)

**Chemoattractant:** A cellular surface receptor that interacts with circulating cytokines to induce inflammatory and immunological function

**Coccygodynia (or coccydynia):** Pain in the region of the coccyx

**Conus medullaris:** The cone-shaped tapering of the lower terminal portion of the spinal cord

**Diathermy:** Shortwave or microwave diathermy is the therapeutic application of high-frequency currents for musculoskeletal pain control

**Dimples of Venus:** Small, natural indentations or pits overlying the posterior superior iliac spines, which is a region that is commonly associated with referred pain in the lumbosacral region

**DISH:** Disseminated idiopathic skeletal hyperostosis. Typically manifested by thickening of the anterior longitudinal ligament bridging its intervertebral portion

**Epidural injection:** Local injections, typically with corticosteroids, into the epidural space for relief of sciatica or spinal stenosis symptoms

**FABERE:** Flexion, abduction, external rotation, extension. Range of motion to test for hip joint pathology

**Facetectomy:** A surgical procedure to remove a portion of the facet joint to relieve neural compression in the root canal

**Fibromyalgia:** A generalized idiopathic non-inflammatory muscle disorder associated with symmetrical areas of focal tenderness in the cervical, dorsal, lumbar and lower extremities, which is often associated with depression, irritable bowel syndrome, migraine and tension headache and may be associated with other connective tissue disorders

**Foot drop gait:** The foot drop (steppage) gait is caused by weakness of dorsiflexion of the foot causing the foot to drop when the leg is raised and to slap down when walking. In the case of sciatica, this is a consequence of primarily L5 nerve root compression

**Interarticular lamina:** Interarticular means between two joints or articulating surfaces. A lamina is a thin, flat layer or membrane, specifically the flattened region of either side of the arch of a vertebra

**Interventional radiology:** Refers to therapeutic procedures performed by a radiologist using various visualization techniques

**Lasègue sign or test:** Test for sciatic nerve irritation performed with the patient supine with knees flexed and feet on the table. The affected leg is then straightened and raised to see if this produces sciatic nerve irritation. A crossed Lasègue test is performed on the opposite leg to see if straight leg raising of the asymptomatic side produces symptoms on the symptomatic side, which is a more precise measure of sciatic nerve irritability

**Litigation neurosis:** Refers to pain and related symptomatology intensified by the legal process and to the potential perpetuation and intensification of pain syndromes and disability, either consciously or otherwise, as a consequence of the psychosomatic stress of a legal process and potential for secondary gain from prolonged or intensified disability

**Manual muscle test:** Muscle strength of various muscle groups is determined by manual resistance applied at specific anatomical regions, e.g. the dorsal surface of the knee to test hip flexors, and is graded 0–5, from total weakness to normal, assuming pain and/or skeletal contractures are not present. Typically, muscle testing is performed on the affected side and then the results compared with those on the normal side

**McKenzie therapy:** A self-treatment concept for disk-related disorders, in which extension postures and/or 'shift correction' sideways slowly-applied mobilization is done to attempt to relieve disk-related neural compression

**Meniscoid:** Pertaining to a crescent (meniscus)-shaped fold of intra-articular facet joint synovium

**MMPI:** Minnesota Multiphasic Personality Inventory. A standard test of psychological function

**Neurogenic claudication:** Lameness or limping as a consequence of impairment of nerve impulses, particularly as a consequence of spinal or nerve root canal stenosis

**Nociceptor:** A peripheral neural structure that is capable of generating nerve impulses in response to painful or injurious stimuli

**Osteochondromatosis:** Benign osseous and/or cartilaginous bodies typically occur near the end of bony (vertebral) and articular structures. Hereditary osteochondromatosis is associated with multiple osteochondromata which more commonly than not are asymptomatic

**Piriformis syndrome:** Sciatic pain caused by compression of the sciatic nerve or a branch of the sciatic nerve by the piriformis muscle, owing to post-traumatic scarring, congenital malformation or focal referred piriformis muscle spasm.

**PMMA:** Poly(methyl methacrylate), a bone-cementing substance that is administered percutaneously into the vertebral body in the treatment of compression fractures

**'Red flags':** Markers of possible systemic disorders that can be causal factors in back pain

**Reiter's syndrome:** Inflammatory arthritis characterized by joint inflammation associated with ankylosing spondylitis, urethritis, diarrhea, conjunctivitis and dermatitis

**RICE:** Rest, ice, corset (brace) and exercise

**Rolfing:** A technique also called 'structural integration' by its inventor, Dr Ida Rolf. The concept is deep fascial massage and often painful manipulation with the purpose of correcting contractures and malalignment

**Romberg test:** Test for balance dysfunction related to cerebellar or vestibular mechanisms and posterior column spinal cord and peripheral neuropathies. The patient stands with the feet close together and then closes his/her eyes. In a positive Romberg test, the patient has no gross imbalance with the eyes open and sways or loses balance when the eyes are closed

**Scheuermann's disease:** Adolescent dorsal epiphyseal aseptic necrosis of the endplates of vertebral bodies (osteochondritis deformans)

**Schmorl's node:** A herniation of the nucleus pulposus through a localized defect in the cartilage-bony endplate of a vertebral body. These commonly occur in the absence of osteoporosis or other possible predisposing factors

**Sciatic scoliosis:** A deviation of the trunk and hence the vertebrae to minimize pressure of a discal protrusion on a nerve root. Scoliosis may be either to the right or the left depending on the position of the discal protrusion and adjacent traumatized nerve root

**Sclerotomes:** The cluster of cells that are the primordial embryonic structures of the vertebral-related tissues

**SEP:** Sensory evoked potentials. Used in electrodiagnosis

**SIP:** Sickness Impact Profile. A measure of the effects of an illness on discomfort and quality of life

**Spina bifida:** A limited defect in the spinal column as a consequence of the absence of the adjacent vertebral arches, through which spinal membranes and rarely the spinal cord may protrude

**Substance P:** A member of a group of peptides (neurokinins) that are neurotransmitters highly concentrated in the dorsal horn where the dorsal horn nociceptors are stimulated by pain. P stands for pain, and in addition to transmission of painful stimuli it may, along with other chemical mediators, contribute to associated soft-tissue inflammatory responses

**Tender point:** A focal area of tenderness on pressure over a bursal area, tendinous insertion or joint

**TENS:** Transcutaneous electrical nerve stimulation

**Trigger point:** A focal area of accentuated muscle tenderness

**VAS:** Visual analog scale. A simple instrument for pain and function monitoring

# Introduction

In parallel with the evolution of the human brain over the last 5 million years, the human skeleton has evolved to liberate us from a quadrupedal gait, and permits us to stand, walk and run with our heads held high in an upright posture. In the enlarged cerebral cortices, a hierarchy of neural centers process thought and action, pain and reaction. Afferent and efferent neural pathways transmitted through the spinal cord dictate and monitor our posture, our gait and all other activities involving our musculoskeletal functions and pain perceptions. Ultimately, however, all that a human being is capable of doing physically depends on the construction of the osseous skeleton and the arrangements and functioning of the supporting ligaments, muscles, tendons and nerves.

In 70% of cases, low back pain has no obvious etiology or pathogenesis, so what makes the back hurt? Most back pain is actually muscular or ligamentous in origin rather than skeletal, and so radiography, including computed tomography (CT), will usually provide no meaningful information, despite the emphasis placed on it by both doctors and society. Ultrasonography or magnetic resonance imaging (MRI), however, may show a soft tissue abnormality. Close clinical examination may often reveal the site of the pathology and the opportunity for cure.

*Fast Facts – Low Back Pain* describes the causes and clinical assessment of low back pain, and aims to provide guidance on making appropriate therapeutic choices to gain optimal relief for each individual back pain patient.

# Therapeutic exercises and protective maneuvers

## Mechanisms of pain

The precise pathophysiological mechanisms involved in pain perception in low back pain disorders are not well understood. When musculoskeletal dysfunction and tissue damage occur, a number of neurohumoral factors may be energized. In the intervertebral disks, a normal anulus fibrosus (but not a normal non-traumatized nucleus pulposus) is highly enervated by pain fibers and capable of provoking a pain response. The same is true of the posterior longitudinal ligament of the spine. Afferent neurons in the dorsal root ganglia stimulate production of substance P, a chemoattractant and vasodilator, and somatostatin, together with other neuropeptides including prostaglandins and leukotrienes. Prostaglandins and leukotrienes are released by activated nociceptors when there is local tissue injury to the anulus and/or adjacent neural, ligamentous and synovial tissues, and play important roles in pain, inflammation, and healing processes. This pain–inflammation reaction can be inhibited by corticosteroids and non-steroidal anti-inflammatory drugs (NSAIDs).

## Psychological factors affecting pain

Any painful stimulus affecting the body is ultimately experienced in the mind. There it is modulated by genetically determined pain transmission and reception capabilities, familial and social conditioning, and increasingly by medicolegal and work-related socioeconomic factors and the possibility of malingering. All of these factors are further modifiable by experiences of previous trauma, surgery and medication, as well as by general and specific health issues. We must therefore not only carefully assess the somatic aspects that have focused the patient's symptoms, and hence our attention, onto the low back, but also relate the demonstrable clinical features to the individual whose back it is.

Back pain is, in the truest sense, psychosomatic. Psychological issues must be addressed concurrently with the anatomic and pathological somatic aspects of low back pain-related disorders. Psychosocial issues must be prioritized, though they can often be readily handled by the patient and the practitioner. If this is not the case, they should be addressed promptly with appropriate psychiatric, psychological and/or social counseling according to need. Issues relating to drug habituation, depression, symptom amplification and chronic pain syndromes must be identified and addressed. As far as possible, pain-relieving strategies must be structured and coordinated to implement a prompt return to family, workplace and social activities.

## Anatomic structures involved in generating pain

Many anatomic factors can play a primary or a secondary role in the development and progression of low back pain syndromes.

**Vertebrae** (cervical, thoracic and lumbar) are designed to perform various functional tasks. The lumbar spine supports the torso and permits flexion, lateral flexion and extension. The facet joint alignments restrict rotation except at the lumbosacral junction, where the heavy iliolumbar ligaments provide restraint. At the junction of the fifth lumbar vertebra and the sacrum, the sacrovertebral angle slopes downward, causing the truncal center of gravity, after passing through the fifth lumbar vertebra, to press on the thick anteriorly wedged fifth lumbar disk. This in turn leads to increased wear and tear on the lower lumbar disks, the adjacent vertebrae and their facet joints, and hence to interarticular laminar deficiencies which predispose the lumbosacral junction and lower lumbar vertebrae to spondylolisthesis.

It should be remembered that a 'pain in the neck' can place a painful burden on the low back. Tenderness and pain at the cervicothoracic junction may often cause the heavy head (5–7 kg) to tilt forward, allowing the center of gravity to change. This adds to the vicious cycle of more pain, worsening posture, more mechanical dysfunction, more muscle spasm and more pain, not only in the neck, but in the low back as well.

*Spondylolisthesis* is perhaps in the truest sense a 'slipped disk' (although the latter term is colloquially applied more generally to any disk protrusion or extrusion). The vertebrae slip over each other, and so the disk must also slip. Pronounced discal slippage may contribute to adjacent nerve root impingement, adding to the spinal canal narrowing already resulting from vertebral overlap, and thereby contributing, along with accompanying facet and degenerative spondylosis, to the potential development of spinal stenosis and to recurrent and chronic low back pain syndromes. Fortunately, the symptoms of spinal stenosis (neurogenic claudication) tend to stabilize and often do not progress. The most common type of spondylolisthesis is anterolisthesis, with the superior vertebra anteriorly overriding the one below, but retrolisthesis and lateral listhesis are also seen, usually as a consequence of intradiscal and secondary facet degenerative pathology occurring in the upper (L2–L3) lumbar vertebrae.

Spondylolisthesis is usually graded in four stages (Figure 1.1), depending on the degree of vertebral slippage:
- grade 1: 25% or less slippage
- grade 2: 25–50% slippage or overlap
- grade 3: 50–75% overlap
- grade 4: the superior vertebra almost completely or completely overrides the lower one.

Even though spondylolisthesis is often not accompanied by low back pain, characteristic findings on examination become increasingly

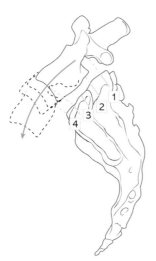

**Figure 1.1** Grades of spondylolisthesis of L5 on S1.

apparent as the graded severity of the spondylolisthesis increases from 1 to 3.

Spondylolisthesis is typically a consequence of bilateral defects (spondylolysis) in the vertebral pars interarticularis, which lead to their separation and hence vertebral slippage. Spondylolysis alone or accompanied by mild spondylolisthesis occurs in about 5% of the adult population, and is generally asymptomatic or associated with only mild low back pain.

These lytic defects are attributed to a congenital failure of bone fusion during maturation, for which there can be a strong familial predisposition. They occur between 5 and 20 years of age, but are usually asymptomatic until later adult life. They may also be a consequence of stress fractures, as they are more common in female gymnasts, male weight-lifters and college football linemen. They have also been attributed to fractures occurring during fetal and neonatal development. Spondylolisthesis of the lower lumbar vertebrae (most common at L5–S1 and less common at L4–L5) can also result from discal and secondary facet degeneration. Spondylolysis is also used to describe stages of age- and trauma-related disk deterioration and, like spondylolisthesis, is graded 1–4.

Hamstring tightness, another predisposing factor for low back pain, is commonly found and may be associated with varying degrees of flexion of the hips and knees on standing, as well as shortening and flattening of the trunk. As the trunk shortens, the waistline widens and side bending is restricted, and when truncal shortening is more pronounced the abdomen protrudes. Even in milder cases, a telltale marker of spondylolisthesis in the form of a protruding hard lump in the midline at the base of the spine may be found. This is the spinous process of the fifth lumbar vertebra, which gains prominence due to forward slippage of the fourth lumbar vertebra caused by anterior spondylolisthesis of L4 over L5.

As spondylolisthesis predisposes to low back stress and strain and the resultant low back pain disorders, confirmation of its presence in symptomatic patients should prompt appropriate conservative treatment; only occasionally is surgical fusion appropriate. It should be remembered, however, that radiological evidence of spondylolisthesis may not be the explanation for the back pain, as major degrees of listhesis can occur without symptoms.

*Other bone pathologies.* A number of other bone pathologies may also cause back pain. They include:

- infective causes, e.g. osteomyelitis and tuberculosis
- neoplastic causes, e.g. primary and secondary tumors, myeloma
- metabolic causes, e.g. osteoporosis and osteomalacia
- idiopathic causes, e.g. Paget's disease and Scheuermann's disease (see page 25).

**Facet (zygapophyseal) joints** (Figure 1.2) are synovial-lined, cartilage-surfaced diarthrodial joints that are connected by a ligamentous joint capsule. Facet joint malalignments and associated degenerative osteoarthritic changes (Figure 1.3) are commonly noted radiographically with or without, and before and after, any accompanying low back pain disorders. This does not preclude an abnormal facet joint being a causal factor of a low back pain syndrome. This can be confirmed by a selective joint injection of hypertonic saline under fluoroscopic visualization to attempt to reproduce the pain, followed by a local anesthetic injection to provide specific relief of the induced pain. The facet joint pain referral pattern thus elicited may not be limited to the lumbar region, and may radiate into the buttock and/or down the leg, mimicking a sciatic nerve root pain.

Osteoarthritic vertebral and facet joint osteophytes, plus facet malalignments and discal protrusions (see Figure 1.4b on page 16), can all predispose to and contribute to a nerve root impingement and

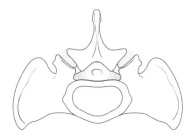

**Figure 1.2** Superior view of facet (zygapophyseal) joints between the inferior articular process of L5 and the superior articular process of S1.

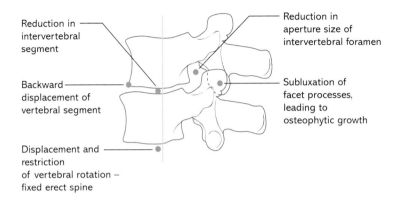

**Figure 1.3** Facet joint malalignment in degenerative disease.

radicular symptoms. Occasionally, a synovial cyst may protrude from an arthritic facet joint and cause compression of an adjacent nerve root.

Some, but not all lumbar facet joints may have intra-articular meniscoid synovial thickenings that are potentially capable of being impinged during stressful lumbar movements, and thereby cause pain. It has been suggested that the release of a meniscal impingement could possibly explain the prompt relief that sometimes occurs with manual manipulation therapies. The audible cracking sound that can be elicited with the instantaneous abrupt facet joint displacement during a manipulation may be attributable to the snapping of an abrupt ligamentous displacement or to the creation of an intra-articular relative vacuum, similar to when a knuckle-cracking manipulation is performed.

**Sacroiliac joints.** The sacroiliac joint (see Figure 1.6 on page 19) was once thought to be the major factor in low back pain and sciatica, but discovery of the role of disk protrusions has dramatically changed that perception. Although there is no question about the role of the sacroiliac joint in the spondyloarthropathies – ankylosing spondylitis, Reiter's syndrome, psoriatic arthritis – and, much less commonly, in infection, tumor or trauma, its role in low back pain and/or sciatic pain referral is questionable. Radiographic evidence of degenerative or malalignment abnormalities of the sacroiliac joints are commonly found, often in the absence of back pain. Evidence supporting the pain referral patterns of lumbar disks and facet joints to the sacroiliac region is irrefutable, but this is not evidence of a causative role for the sacroiliac joint in a low back pain syndrome. Despite the variety of examination procedures designed to confirm the presence of sacroiliac pathology, most notably subluxations potentially amenable to manipulation or other therapy, there is no consistent reproducibility of the various methods when careful assessments have been made by blinded experts. Even in ankylosing spondylitis, invariably associated with sacroiliitis, the localization of sacroiliac pain remains unclear. This uncertainty about the role of the sacroiliac joint and the difficulty in establishing a firm diagnosis of sacroiliac pathology is reflected in the scant mention made of it in current texts on low back pain.

Conservative management of lumbar and lumbosacral painful disorders can usually be successfully undertaken without specifically addressing the sacroiliac joint per se. Nevertheless, non-inflammatory symptomatic sacroiliac derangements do occur, and can be confirmed by fluoroscopically guided local injections. A local corticosteroid injection can provide a useful therapeutic option in the few patients in whom the diagnosis is confirmed. The role of manipulation therapy in resolving a specific sacroiliac derangement is questionable, but to discount it totally would cause great consternation to the many who have been convinced by their experience (placebo or otherwise) of its benefits.

*Sacralization/lumbaralization* of the lumbosacral vertebrae, and/or various degrees of fusion of transverse processes, are not per se typically associated with low back pain, though they may contribute to restricted lumbar movement and secondary strain.

**Disks and their associated ligaments** are designed to absorb shock and simultaneously to transmit imposed forces in many directions. This is made possible by the resistive quality of the fluid contained in the nucleus pulposus, coupled with the elasticity of the surrounding anulus fibrosus. The fluidity of the nucleus pulposus resists primarily vertical

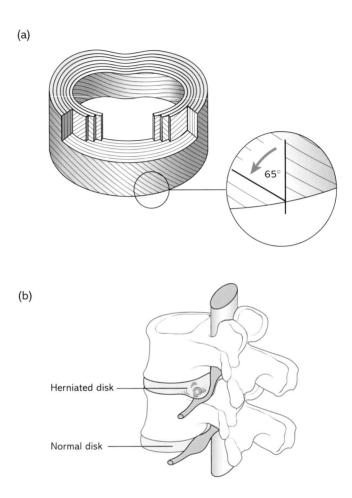

**Figure 1.4** Intervertebral disk structure and pathology: (a) orientation of collagen fibers in a lumbar anulus fibrosus; (b) herniated disk.

compressive forces, and distributes them radially into the anulus fibrosus, which is uniquely designed with alternating bands of fibers to resist torsional strains (Figure 1.4a). Despite these design features, however, disks do wear, tear, rupture, protrude and extrude, though fortunately they usually heal. The consequences of disk herniations (Figure 1.4b) range from none (asymptomatic) to agonizing pain and paresis.

The posterior longitudinal ligamentous constraints are weaker posterolaterally, and so most disk protrusions occur away from the midline and may impact the laterally placed nerve roots. Because of the more vertical alignment of the lower nerve roots in the cauda equina, the fifth lumbar nerve roots will be vulnerable to impaction by a posterolateral protrusion of the fourth lumbar disk (see posterior longitudinal ligament below).

**Other ligaments** (Figure 1.5) are the following.

*The ligamenta flava* consist of yellowish elastic fibers distributed vertically between the laminar arches, permitting extension without in-folding and pinching compression of the nerve tissue. The intertransverse ligaments lie deep to the tendinous insertions of the

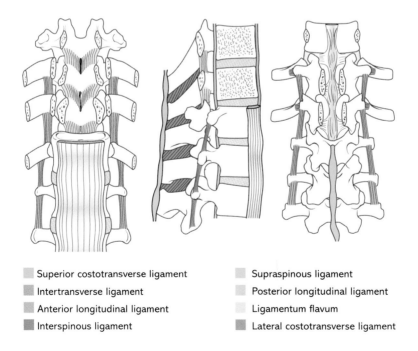

　Superior costotransverse ligament

　Intertransverse ligament

　Anterior longitudinal ligament

　Interspinous ligament

　Supraspinous ligament

　Posterior longitudinal ligament

　Ligamentum flavum

　Lateral costotransverse ligament

**Figure 1.5** Spinal ligaments.

segmental muscles on the transverse processes. The interspinous ligaments bridge between the spinous processes beneath the longer and heavier, overlying, supraspinous ligament.

*The anterior longitudinal ligament* is a heavy ligament that blends firmly with the periosteum of the vertebral body, and is loosely attached to the anterior aspect of the anulus. It is most firmly attached to the articular lip, or rim, of each vertebral body, thus accounting for the occurrence of so-called traction spurs and rim osteophytes (spurs) as a consequence of discal dysfunctions and ligamentous strains.

*The posterior longitudinal ligament*, in contrast, is not attached to the vertebral body. It is bow-strung over the concave posterior surface of the vertebra, leaving space for the vascular elements to enter and leave the medullary sinuses. The strong mid-portion of the posterior longitudinal ligament tends to resist annular protrusion, but as noted above, disk protrusions can more easily penetrate laterally.

**Bursae.** The function of all bursae (see Figure 1.6) is to minimize the potential for friction as a consequence of a muscle rubbing normally on a bony prominence. The bursae can be overloaded, however, and become inflamed. Bursitis associated with low back pain and hip joint arthritis usually originates at the submaximus trochanteric bursa and, less often, at the obturator internis bursa. The submaximus bursa is of particular interest because it is not uncommonly associated with a sciatic-like, neuralgic pain referred to the lateral thigh. The precise basis for the development of trochanteric bursitis is not always apparent, though it appears to be related to reflex-induced tension of the muscles that pass over the bursa occurring as a consequence of referred lumbar disk-related pain, or to torsional strain as a consequence of gait alterations in the case of hip and/or knee joint disorders, or leg length asymmetry.

Bursitis is associated with focal tenderness on palpation with moderate pressure over the anatomic location of the bursa in question. Bursal tenderness of the subgluteus-medius bursa is less common. Ischiogluteal bursitis, which usually results from trauma to or pressure on and irritation of an ischial tuberosity, is otherwise unrelated to low back discogenic disorders.

**Paraspinal muscles.** The paraspinal musculature, which is essential to postural stabilization and mobilization of the trunk, consists of two main types.

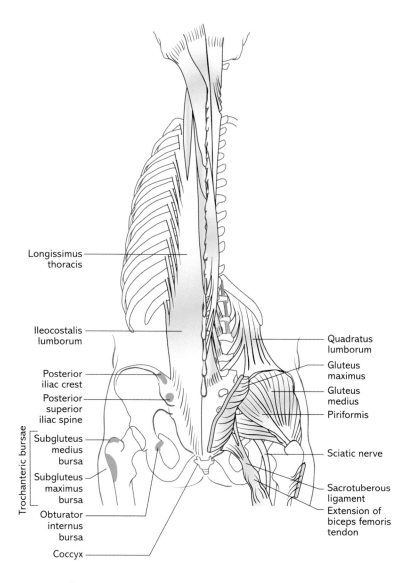

Figure 1.6 Some anatomic structures involved in the development of low back pain.

19

- The small muscle group consists of two short intersegmental muscles: the interspinalis muscles that bridge the spinous processes and the intertransversarii that bridge the transverse processes.
- The multifidus and erector spinae form two large, polysegmental muscle groups.

The multifidus is the most medial. Its origin is on the spinous processes, with insertions on the vertebral mamillary processes, the posterior superior iliac spine, the dorsal aspect of the sacrum, and the posterior sacroiliac ligament. The erector spinae consists primarily of the longissimus thoracis and the ileocostalis lumborum with a third small component, the spinalis dorsi, which only attaches to the spinous processes of L1, L2 and L3. The erector spinae muscles originate on the lower ribs and thoracic transverse processes and insert on the lumbar vertebrae, the iliac crests and adjacent to the posterior superior iliac spines.

Although muscle 'spasm' of the erector spinae in association with acute pain is common, pain referral and muscle spasm with focal tenderness (a trigger point) in the mid-portion of the quadratus lumborum muscle and/or a tender point on the mid-iliac crest is more often noted. This can be a consequence of pain referral from vertebral facet or discal strains at either the dorsolumbar origins or the ileolumbar insertions of the erector spinae muscles.

**The gluteal and piriformis muscles** are shown in Figure 1.6. The primary functions of the gluteal muscles are to support, stabilize and mobilize the hips and lower extremities in relation to the pelvis and the trunk. Possibly the most common manifestation of lumbar and lumbosacral pain referral is to the mid-portion of the gluteal muscles (buttocks) that overlie the piriformis muscle. This is accompanied by a palpable localized region of deep, tender muscle induration. Because of the thickness of the overlying gluteus maximus muscle, whose fibers are parallel to (and indistinguishable from) the piriformis muscle fibers, it is not possible to determine by palpation if the piriformis muscle per se is the source of the localized muscle tenderness. A 'piriformis syndrome' is therefore somewhat problematic to identify and must be carefully distinguished from the more common, spinal discogenic basis for sciatic radiculopathy. A piriformis syndrome may result from scarring after a fall on the buttocks or as a consequence of pelvic or hip surgeries. MRI can be used to visualize the tender area in the buttocks and help to identify selective piriformis entrapments of the sciatic nerve.

**Lumbar nerves** transmit the stimuli for all sensory and motor functions in the lower extremities, though previous or concomitant central or peripheral nervous system disorders may also affect sensation, balance and coordination.

The spinal cord terminates in the conus medullaris at the upper border of the second lumbar vertebra. Nerve roots in the lumbosacral spine consist of a posterior or dorsal root with afferent sensory fibers and the dorsal root ganglia, and an anterior or ventral root with efferent motor fibers. These anterior and posterior roots fuse, and the nerve roots thus formed in the dorsolumbar region descend almost vertically to form the cauda equina before exiting through their respective nerve root canals. The sensory fibers consist of:

- large, rapidly conducting type A fibers that transmit touch, pressure and proprioception
- smaller, more slowly conducting type B fibers that transmit pain and temperature
- small unmyelinated type C pain-transmitting fibers.

The sensory neural components of the nerve roots enervate their respective peripheral nerves, sclerotomes and dermatomes (see Figure 2.12 on page 50). Each dermatome is innervated by a specific nerve root, but there is considerable overlap between the dermatomes and considerable variation between individuals. Most radiculopathies, and particularly those associated with low back pain and sciatica, are the result of disk-related nerve root compressions (Figure 1.7). The extent of clinical manifestations of radiculopathy related to apparently similar nerve root compressions, e.g. the same disk levels and apparently similar herniations, is also variable. Nerve root compression can cause sensory impairment, less often both sensory and motor nerve root impairment, and occasionally only motor nerve root dysfunction, e.g. a foot drop gait or demonstrable weakness on physical

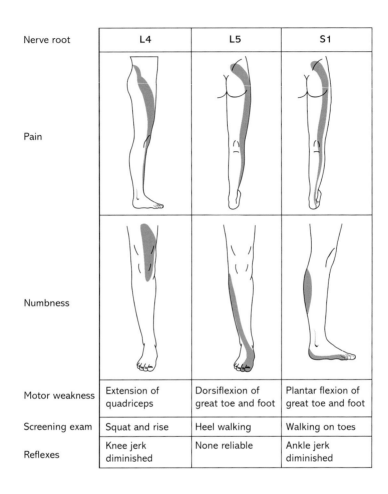

| Nerve root | L4 | L5 | S1 |
|---|---|---|---|
| Motor weakness | Extension of quadriceps | Dorsiflexion of great toe and foot | Plantar flexion of great toe and foot |
| Screening exam | Squat and rise | Heel walking | Walking on toes |
| Reflexes | Knee jerk diminished | None reliable | Ankle jerk diminished |

**Figure 1.7** Syndromes of the most common radiculopathies, involving disk compression of the nerve roots at L4, L5 or S1.

examination. The extent and severity of neural dysfunction is related to the degree of neural compression and its duration.

Cells within the dorsal root ganglia process painful stimuli with the resultant release of substance P and other neuropeptides within the dorsal column of the spinal cord. The sympathetic afferent fibers in the lumbar region enter the four to six sensory sympathetic ganglia along each side of the anterior vertebral column and subsequently enter the spinal cord via the ventral nerve root. Afferent sympathetic fibers interface with cells in the dorsal root ganglia, while efferent fibers emanate from the sympathetic ganglia and are then distributed in conjunction with the sensory and motor nerve fibers to the various sympathetic effectors, e.g. blood vessels and sweat glands. Axons of the post-ganglionic sympathetic fibers are the only autonomic adrenergic fibers that interact with α-receptors (skin and muscle vasoconstriction with cold, stress or Raynaud's phenomenon) and β-receptors (sweating to cool and vasodilation to enhance vascular flow to maintain muscular function and body temperature during exercise).

Compression of nerve roots or ganglia per se does not cause pain, but does impair both sensory and motor functioning. Compression in association with inflammation and congestion of the nerve roots and/or ganglia, as well as adjacent ligamentous and articular tissues, however, does cause release of substance P and other pain-stimulating cytokines.

Sensory dysfunctions resulting from disk–nerve-root disorders usually manifest in a fairly specific dermatomal pattern. Sclerotomal, or deep pain, referral patterns are more diffuse and do not follow the classic dermatomes. Concomitant specific nerve impairment from previous or associated disorders can make the clinical assessment of nerve root impairment on a lumbar discogenic basis more difficult and may necessitate additional electrodiagnostic and other testing. The L1–L2 disk is seldom affected in low back discal disorders, so compression of the conus medullaris is a 'red flag' (see Table 2.1 on page 33) not only because of the severe nature of the neurologic complications but also because of the likelihood of malignancy as the cause.

**Vascular components.** For practical purposes, the circulation to the spine is not a concern unless a surgical procedure is undertaken, or possibly if a clot in an artery causes avascular necrosis.

The segmental arterial supply to the lumbar vertebrae and adjacent muscles consists of paired arteries that branch off the posterior surface of the aorta. The dorsum of each vertebra is supplied by the four arteries from two adjacent vertebrae that have entered through the intervertebral foramina. The venous system consists largely of a complex of valveless, cross-connected, epidural channels that drain into the intercostal and lumbar veins. In addition to venous drainage, these epidural venous channels can also provide a shock-absorbing cushion to protect the spinal cord and cauda equina.

## Congenital and developmental abnormalities

Although the spine is very cleverly designed and very adaptable, it contains many structural subtleties that predispose it to the consequences of wear and tear and trauma. In addition, it is not always congenitally fabricated properly, nor does it always develop correctly during growth.

**Ligaments, tendons and fascias.** Our genes dictate our individual human identities, including our musculoskeletal and neural structures, vascular tissues, immune systems and responsiveness to inflammation and trauma. The ligaments and tendons of the musculoskeletal system are highly varied structures, each individually designed to perform a specific task. The universal assignment for the ligaments is to hold the various skeletal structures together. Some ligaments, such as the anterior longitudinal ligaments, are thick, firm and unyielding. Others, such as the ligamenta flava, contain elastic fibers designed to permit a wide range of motion and suppleness. All ligaments, tendons and fascias, however, are designed to impose specific constraints while facilitating purposeful movements of a specific anatomic region.

Normal ligaments, tendons and fascias respond to physical stresses without undue strain, though there is a considerable range of flexibility within what is considered normal in these tissues. For example, both increased ligamentous laxity (simple double-jointedness or benign joint hypermobility syndrome) and more profound collagen defective disorders (e.g. Ehlers–Danlos syndrome or Marfan's syndrome) increase vulnerability to joint and spinal wear and tear, subluxations and degenerative changes, presumably as a consequence of the less restrictive ligaments permitting joints to be more readily traumatized during activities of daily living. Often this is compounded by the vigorous stretching maneuvers, e.g. yoga, ballet or gymnastics, encouraged by the joint laxity. Such ligamentous laxity is associated with a tendency to scoliosis that may be complicated by vertebral

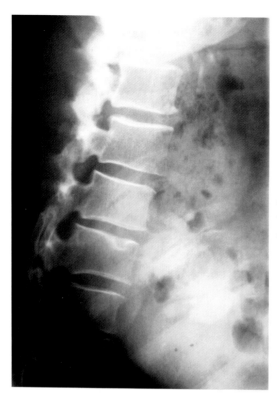

**Figure 1.8**
Scheuermann's disease:
avascular necrosis of
the apophyseal rings of
vertebral bodies.

abnormalities, and to spondylolisthesis with consequent facet
arthropathies and/or spinal stenosis.

**Scheuermann's disease** (osteochondromatosis or juvenile kyphosis)
(Figure 1.8) occurs spontaneously during adolescence at the time of
rapid growth and development. It is more common in females than in
males. Pathological alteration and necrosis of the cartilage and bone
of the vertebral end-plate result in end-plate irregularities during the
healing phase. Schmorl's nodes, disk space narrowing, anterior wedging
and occasional intervertebral fusions are readily demonstrated by
radiography. Scheuermann's disease may be asymptomatic or associated
with varying degrees of discomfort and kyphotic deformity. The apex of
the kyphotic curve is typically at T7–T9, and it is therefore sometimes
confused with, or can occur in association with, kyphosis resulting
from osteoporotic fractures.

**Spina bifida** is seldom associated with low back pain, but it has been associated with compression of the unprotected nerve roots in the cauda equina, which can occur during vigorous lumbar extension in the absence of the bony laminae that normally provide a protective cover.

## Spinal rigidity

Any structural alteration or congenital abnormality that restricts intervertebral movement inevitably imposes a greater mechanical stress on higher and lower discal and vertebral segments that have retained movement capability. This predisposes the moveable disk's annular and adjacent ligaments, and the end-plates and facet joints, to greater wear and tear, more rapid degeneration, and secondary arthrosis.

Rigidity of vertebral segments can result from congenital, post-traumatic or surgical fusions (Figure 1.9), or from degenerative disk

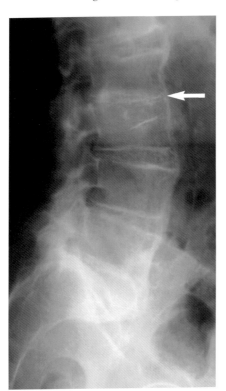

**Figure 1.9** Lumbar fusion causing spinal rigidity. There is obvious anterior longitudinal ligament bony fusion. The arrow indicates bony bridging anteriorly between vertebrae.

shrinkage and secondary osteophyte formation. Ankylosing spondylitis and disseminated idiopathic skeletal hyperostosis (DISH) can restrict spinal movement segmentally as well as diffusely, depending on the extent of the longitudinal and periannular ligamentous ossification and fusion and any associated muscle spasm. Where movement between vertebrae does occur, additional wear and tear strains are imposed on the remaining mobile osseous vertebral and ligamentous segments. Examination will reveal restricted movement and a flattened lumbar curve.

## Spinal stenosis

Morphological spinal stenosis (Figure 1.10) and/or root foraminal stenosis, with consequent disturbance of neural function, can be congenital, associated with spondylolisthesis (see page 10), secondary to discal protrusions, ligamentous thickening and ossifications, or any combination of these factors. Not uncommonly, spinal stenosis identified radiographically during differential diagnosis of a low back pain syndrome is considered to be the cause of the pain. Although this is a possibility, the stenosis is more likely to be simply an associated phenomenon, comparable to noting the presence of an osteophyte in the same or an adjacent area.

Clinically significant spinal stenosis is characterized by neurogenic (pseudo) claudication, but the symptoms of neurogenic claudication are not invariably associated with low back pain. Similar but unilateral symptoms may be caused by nerve root canal stenosis. The classic clinical symptoms of neurogenic claudication are heaviness and aching, with or without dysesthesias or numbness, in the thighs and lower legs brought on by standing erect or walking for varying periods of time and promptly relieved (within 2–5 minutes) by sitting or lying down, and sometimes by just leaning forward. Vascular claudication, in contrast, is typically relieved by simply standing still, as well as by sitting or lying down, to restore adequate circulation. The symptoms of neurogenic claudication that result from spinal stenosis are caused by neural compression in the cauda equinal or specific nerve root canals when the spinal canal or specific root canals are constricted in the upright posture. Neurogenic

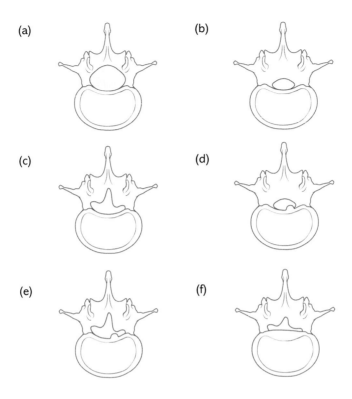

**Figure 1.10** Lumbar spinal stenosis: (a) normal vertebral canal; (b) congenital/developmental stenosis; (c) degenerative stenosis; (d) congenital/developmental stenosis with disk herniation; (e) degenerative stenosis with disk herniation; (f) congenital/developmental stenosis with superimposed degenerative stenosis.

claudication depends on time and posture, but not on activity or energy utilization.

Although patients with spinal stenosis may complain of back discomfort and/or stiffness or pain with changing position or with activity, these are manifestations of associated lumbar or lumbosacral pathologies, and are not due to the spinal stenosis per se. Examination of lower extremity pulses, particularly the dorsalis pedis and posterior tibial pulses, can help diagnose vascular claudication, but both spinal stenosis and arteriosclerosis can occur in the same patient. Spinal stenosis is most often a geriatric problem, and it can be symptomatically compounded by or confused with a number of conditions, including:

- peripheral arteriosclerosis
- current or previous sciatica
- osteoarthritis of hips or knees
- peripheral neuropathies
- Paget's disease
- spinal cord tumors.

A clear differential diagnosis of clinical lumbar spinal stenosis is therefore dependent on more than radiographic confirmation. Clinical features relating to pain and functional impairment, and careful neurological assessment, should be taken into consideration before proceeding with aggressive surgical interventions, unless the development of bowel, bladder, sexual or motor dysfunction dictates a need for urgent surgical intervention.

## Traumatic factors

**Fractures.** Lumbar fractures are usually related to trauma and quite straightforward to diagnose. Atraumatic vertebral compression fractures as a result of severe osteoporosis are not uncommon, however, and may be associated with minimal or no pain. Such non-malignant, osteoporotic fractures seldom occur in the cervical spine and are also less often observed in the lower lumbar vertebrae than in the thoracic and upper lumbar spine.

*Coccygodynia*, pain in the coccygeal region, can be caused by fracture or sprain of the coccyx (see Figure 1.6 on page 19), resulting from trauma, usually a hard fall in a half-seated position with a significant impact on the sacrococcygeal tissues rather than just the ischial tuberosities. Coccygodynia can also result from childbirth trauma or perianal dysfunction, and can be referred pain from lower mid-line disk protrusions. The onset of pain can be acute, with tenderness primarily localized to the coccyx and lower sacrum. Pain is typically brought on by sitting or changing position. Tenderness on palpation of the coccygeal area may also be due to inflammation of the small overlying subcutaneous coccygeal bursa. Sacrococcygeal pain can often be very simply relieved with a single, well placed injection of corticosteroid with an anesthetic.

Non-traumatic coccygodynia, particularly when elicited not by palpation but by motion of the coccyx, can be a manifestation of inflammation of the sacral plexus or of diseases or tumors of the pelvic tissues.

**Soft tissue injuries.** The most important traumatic factors in low back pain relate to soft tissue structures. Precise identification of the injured tissue, and the role of that injury in the consequent pain and dysfunction, can be frustratingly difficult. The tissues most often involved are the ligaments, facet joints, disks and nerve roots. In flexion, the anterior annular fibers are compressed and the posterior fibers stretched. Eighty percent of torsional stress is shared by the anulus and the facet joints. The facet joints are separated in flexion, placing more strain on the anulus and increasing the risk of discal rupture. With age or after a previous injury, the nucleus becomes stiffer, the anulus loses elasticity, and the susceptibility to discal injury is increased. When a neurological dysfunction is detected, the affected nerve root level can usually be identified, but the exact source of the neural impingement and/or trauma may be more elusive.

Healing of any injured tissue is a three-phase process:
- resolution of the acutely traumatized tissue site, e.g. reabsorption of local edema, hemorrhage and damaged tissue debris
- repair of the injured tissues
- remodeling of the damaged tissue, to the extent that this is possible.

The first two processes will inevitably take place, but the end result of the remodeling process can leave the tissues mechanically and functionally impaired.

Pain may also be referred to the spine from other soft tissue injuries, such as:
- vascular injuries, e.g. aortic aneurysm or aortic dissection
- renal injury, e.g. carcinoma or calculus
- gynecologic injury, e.g. uterine carcinoma, pelvic inflammatory disease or endometriosis
- pancreatic disorders, e.g. tumor or pancreatitis.

## Causes of low back pain – Key points

- All back pain is 'psychosomatic', because any somatic pain that is experienced must be experienced in the psyche and then processed by the individual to express its impact.
- Radiographic spinal stenosis, facet arthrosis and disk protrusions are very common and correlate poorly with symptoms after age 50.
- Piriformis tenderness is an area of local tenderness deep to the gluteus maximus muscle, and tenderness palpated in that area most often represents a referred trigger point in the gluteus maximus muscle rather than specific piriformis sciatic nerve syndrome involvement.
- Facet arthritis and trochanteric bursal irritation both may produce symptomatology that mimics sciatic nerve involvement.

## Key references

Cailliet R. Miscellaneous low back conditions relating to pain and disability. In: *Low Back Pain Syndrome*, 5th edn. Philadelphia: FA Davis, 1995.

Calin A, Taurog J, eds. *The Spondylarthritides*. Oxford: Oxford University Press, 1998.

Guanciale A, Dillin W, Watkins R. Back pain in children and adolescents. In: Herkowitz HN, Garfin SR, Balderston RA et al., eds. *Rothman–Simeone: The Spine*, 4th edn. Philadelphia: WB Saunders, 1999:187–220.

Swezey RL, ed. Low Back Pain. *Phys Med Rehabil Clin N Am* 1998;9:309–523.

Wiesel SW, Weinstein JN, Herkowitz H et al., eds. Lumbar spinal stenosis. Ch 9 in: *The Lumbar Spine*, 2nd edn. Philadelphia: ISSLS / WB Saunders, 1996:711–81.

The first encounter with the low back pain patient offers a good opportunity to observe the patient's behavior and gait as they enter the room, get up and down from a chair and then walk to the examination room. If not already completed in the waiting room or before the appointment, it is also possible for the patient to fill out the necessary administrative paper work, a personal and family history form, and complete a pain drawing and a pain intensity assessment (see below). Many observations can be made as the patient moves about the room, transfers from a chair, dresses and undresses, and gets on and off the examination table.

The extent of the inquiry should be appropriate to the severity and chronicity of the back pain problem and should aim to identify relevant confounding factors, including systemic diseases, activities of daily living, work environment, recreation as well as psychological and litigation issues, smoking, and alcohol and analgesic abuse. It is important to have the patient sufficiently undressed to be examined adequately both on the initial visit and, as appropriate, at follow-up visits, so that potentially relevant factors, e.g. varicosities and edema, muscle atrophy, and scarring (including spinal surgical scars), are not overlooked. Time and resources are limiting factors, however, and both must be used efficiently and judiciously. For example, a young healthy adult with an acute back strain, no sciatic symptoms, and only moderate pain can be interviewed and examined much more briefly.

The initial examination also provides an opportunity to observe inappropriate findings of exaggerated grunts, inability to straight leg raise while lying supine but with ability to sit up from a lying position, or other features suggesting psychological overlay or 'litigation neurosis'.

### 'Red flags'

The presence of any of the 'red flags', suggesting serious conditions, detailed in Table 2.1 should be noted at the initial assessment, as they

TABLE 2.1

'Red flags' suggesting serious conditions

| Condition | Findings from medical history | Findings from physical examination |
|---|---|---|
| Possible fracture | • Major trauma, such as vehicle accident or fall from height<br>• Minor trauma or even strenuous lifting, in older or potentially osteoporotic patients | |
| Possible tumor or infection | • Age > 50 or < 20<br>• History of cancer<br>• Constitutional symptoms, such as recent fever or chills or unexplained weight loss<br>• Risk factors for spinal infection, recent bacterial infection (e.g. UTI), intravenous drug use, or immune suppression (from corticosteroid use, transplant or HIV infection)<br>• Pain worse in supine position; severe night-time pain | |
| Possible cauda equina syndrome | • Saddle anesthesia<br>• Recent onset of bladder dysfunction, such as urinary retention, increased frequency, or overflow incontinence<br>• Severe or progressive neurological deficit in the lower extremity | • Unexpected laxity of anal sphincter<br>• Perianal/perineal sensory loss<br>• Major motor weakness: quadriceps (knee extension weakness), ankle plantar flexors, evertors and dorsiflexors (foot drop) |

UTI, urinary tract infection

will influence subsequent management of the back pain. In addition, rare disorders such as acromegaly or ochronosis, or rare manifestations of relatively common diseases such as gout, can very occasionally affect the spinal structures.

## Personal and family history

This should include issues relating to prior low back and other orthopedic problems, and injuries as well as other illnesses. Current and previous treatments and medications used for back pain and their success or failure as well as any side-effects should be listed. The response to any previous therapies is likely to influence a patient's attitude to further management efforts, and in that regard it should be remembered that many, if not most, patients are today being guided by friends, family, advertisements, complementary health practitioners and the internet, not to mention a variety of traditional allopathic specialists or even lawyers.

## Pain intensity

It is usually very helpful to have the patient fill out a brief history and system-review questionnaire, and complete a pain drawing. A simple measure of pain intensity can be obtained using the visual analog scale (VAS). The VAS measures pain on a horizontal 10-cm line, where 0 is no pain and 10 cm is the greatest pain ever (Figure 2.1). The VAS can be repeated at subsequent visits to monitor progress. A pain drawing is also useful in determining the pattern of the pain and possibly its etiology (Figure 2.2). These two assessments are the simplest, least time-dependent and least threatening of the tests available.

More detailed assessments of functional ability and of the patient's perception of the pain and its impact on his/her physical, psychological and socioeconomic functioning can be obtained using any of a large number of questionnaires of varying complexity, including:

- the Oswestry Low Back Pain Disability Questionnaire (ten brief questions, each with six possible answers)
- the Quebec Back Pain Disability Scale (20 short questions scored 0–5 relating to pain, disability and psychological state)

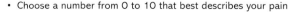

• Choose a number from 0 to 10 that best describes your pain

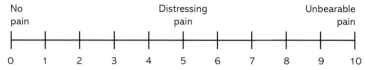

• How much pain have you had because of your condition IN THE PAST WEEK? Place a mark on the line below to indicate how severe your pain has been:

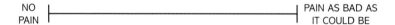

**Figure 2.1** Examples of visual analog scales allowing patients to describe the degree of their pain.

• the Roland–Morris Disability Questionnaire (24 questions plus a five-point vertical 'pain thermometer' also rating pain, disability and psychological state) (Table 2.2).

These three assessments can also be used to monitor progress.

## Pain duration

In the absence of 'red flags' (see Table 2.1) or intractable pain, the clinical evaluation should be responsive not only to the severity of the pain, neurological deficits and concomitant incapacitation, but also to the duration of the symptoms. For the purposes of diagnostic and management decisions, an episode of low back pain can be considered:

• acute, if it has lasted for less than 4 weeks
• subacute, if it has lasted for 4–12 weeks
• chronic, if it has lasted for more than 12 weeks.

All of the initial observations and many more must be made with reference to the duration of the patient's symptoms.

## Psychological assessment

Psychological factors can be of no consequence or play the major role in determining the patient's outcome and return to functional activity. The more chronic the low back pain disorder, the greater the impact of

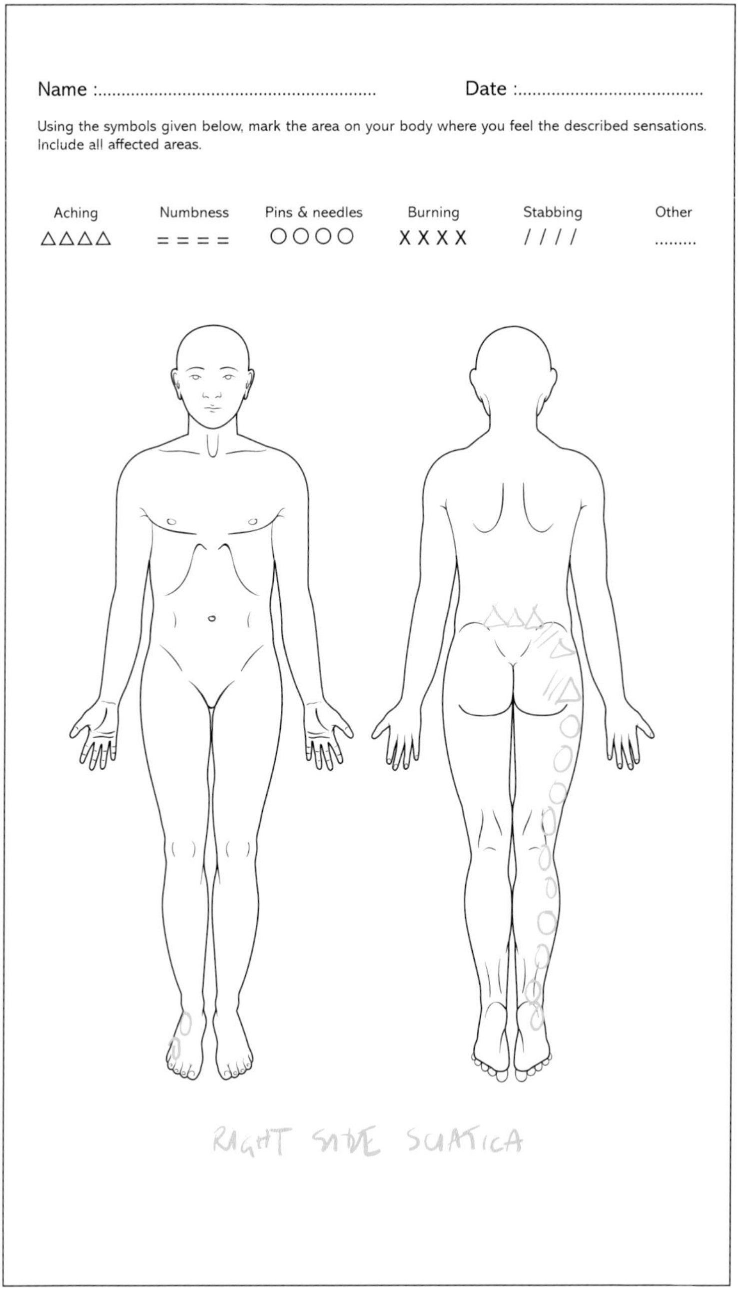

Name :.......................................................          Date :......................................

Using the symbols given below, mark the area on your body where you feel the described sensations. Include all affected areas.

| Aching | Numbness | Pins & needles | Burning | Stabbing | Other |
|--------|----------|----------------|---------|----------|-------|
| △△△△ | = = = = | ○○○○ | X X X X | / / / / | ......... |

RIGHT SIDE SCIATICA

**Figure 2.2** Example of a pain drawing for a patient with right S1 sciatica.

TABLE 2.2

## The Roland–Morris disability questionnaire

Patient name: _____     File # _____ Date: _____

Please read instructions: when your back hurts, you may find it difficult to do some of the things you normally do. Mark only the sentences that describe you today.

[ ]   I stay at home most of the time because of my back.

[ ]   I change position frequently to try to get my back comfortable.

[ ]   I walk more slowly than usual because of my back.

[ ]   Because of my back, I am not doing any jobs that I usually do around the house.

[ ]   Because of my back, I use a handrail to get upstairs.

[ ]   Because of my back, I lie down to rest more often.

[ ]   Because of my back, I have to hold on to something to get out of an easy chair.

[ ]   Because of my back, I try to get other people to do things for me.

[ ]   I get dressed more slowly than usual because of my back.

[ ]   I only stand up for short periods of time because of my back.

[ ]   Because of my back, I try not to bend or kneel down.

[ ]   I find it difficult to get out of a chair because of my back.

[ ]   My back is painful almost all of the time.

[ ]   I find it difficult to turn over in bed because of my back.

[ ]   My appetite is not very good because of my back.

[ ]   I have trouble putting on my socks (or stockings) because of the pain in my back.

[ ]   I can only walk short distances because of my back pain.

[ ]   I sleep less well because of my back.

[ ]   Because of my back pain, I get dressed with the help of someone else.

[ ]   I sit down for most of the day because of my back.

[ ]   I avoid heavy jobs around the house because of my back.

[ ]   Because of back pain, I am more irritable and bad tempered with people than usual.

[ ]   Because of my back, I go upstairs more slowly than usual.

[ ]   I stay in bed most of the time because of my back.

Score: _____ Improvement: _____ %

psychological factors is likely to be. A variety of tests can be used to categorize and document personality and cognitive-behavioral functioning, e.g. whether the patient manifests inappropriate symptom amplification or other psychological disorders. One of the most widely used instruments for this purpose is the Minnesota Multiphasic Personality Inventory (MMPI). This is a comprehensive psychological test that characterizes hypochondriasis, depression and hysteria. The MMPI is useful in identifying psychological disorders that may accompany and complicate back pain and other organic diseases.

Although psychological assessment is often carried out as an integral part of the clinical evaluation of the patient, further more detailed assessment may be indicated.

### Gait assessment

Gait can be assessed more fully, and with the patient less self-conscious, during movement from one room to another, but when patients are fully dressed, some important observations may be obscured. Most obvious is a pain avoidance stride, permitting only brief weight-bearing on the affected side. A gait alteration due to a short leg, or a pronated foot, may also be less evident when the patient is clothed.

*Shuffling* may due to back pain avoidance, hip, knee and foot arthritis, peripheral neuropathy, Parkinson's disease, cardiac, cerebral or peripheral arteriosclerosis, spinal stenosis, visual impairment, or to generalized debility and non-specific pain avoidance with depression and exhaustion.

*Use of a walking stick.* If a walking stick (cane) is used, it should be an appropriate length (neither too long nor too short) to allow for a 20–30° flexion of the elbow when the stick is held at the side. A walking stick with a too smooth rubber tip leaves a patient vulnerable to slipping on wet surfaces. It is also important to observe whether the walking stick is held correctly in the hand opposite the painful side.

*Limping.* A limp favoring only one leg is a common consequence of low back pain, particularly when it is associated with neural impairment and lower extremity weakness. However, a unilateral limp can also be due to arthritis of the foot, ankle, knee or hip, pes planus (flat foot), Morton's neuralgia, or hemiparesis, among other conditions.

*Footwear.* High-heeled and/or loose-fitting shoes should be noted and the patient made aware of possible painful consequences of inadequate foot support.

## Ergonomic awareness

Both the office and the examining room offer excellent opportunities to observe and instruct on ergonomic awareness. If the patient experiences difficulty in sitting or rising from a chair or the examining table, or unnecessarily stoops, twists, reaches, lifts, or carries heavy objects (tools, briefcase, purse, coat and clothing), they can be made aware of the unnecessary stresses and strains they might be incurring and how these might be reduced. Similarly, a patient should be made aware of how to use the body when undressing and dressing. This is also an opportunity to discuss bed positions, pillows and mattresses, and other practical alternatives, e.g. the use of elastic shoelaces or long-handled shoehorns.

## Spinal alignment and movement

The many factors that determine the spine's alignment and movement should be carefully documented, in an attempt to determine the relative contributions of spinal structure and pain to any malalignment noted.

- Structural factors (e.g. scoliosis or a leg length discrepancy) are persistent and basically not pain-dependent contributors.
- Pain is a variable contributor, depending on its intensity and the patient's movement.

Pain avoidance postures can accentuate structural factors, as in the kyphosis resulting from an osteoporotic thoracic spinal fracture. A sciatic scoliosis may be a pain avoidance positioning, as when a disk protrusion impacts on a nerve root when the body leans toward it, in which case it is seen typically during flexion and/or side bending (Figure 2.3). Equally, however, it may result from a mechanically imposed malalignment as a consequence of a disk protrusion creating an intradiscal wedge that tilts the trunk. The typical clinical features of a herniated lumbar disk at L3–L4, L4–L5 or L5–S1 are shown in Figure 2.4.

Spinal malalignment can also be the result of postural adaptations for the avoidance of the discomfort associated with painful lower extremity disorders, e.g. arthritis of the hip or knee.

**Examination pointers.** A number of useful observations can be made in relation to spinal alignment and the localization of pain (Table 2.3). Any of these patterns may indicate the location and possible nature of the pain-provoking lesion, but with the possible exception of a specific radicular pain associated with a corresponding sensory deficit, none has sufficient specificity to make a definitive diagnosis.

(a)

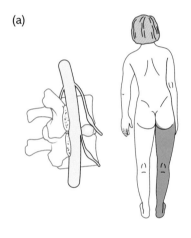

(b)

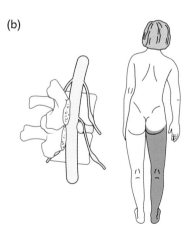

**Figure 2.3** Sciatic scoliosis. A herniated nucleus pulposus is causing ipsilateral leg pain (shaded leg). In (a) the patient lists to the contralateral side to relieve compression of the nerve by the herniated disk. In (b) the patient lists to the ipsilateral side to relieve tenting of the nerve over the herniated disk.

| Level of herniation | Pain | Numbness | Weakness | Atrophy | Reflexes |
|---|---|---|---|---|---|
| 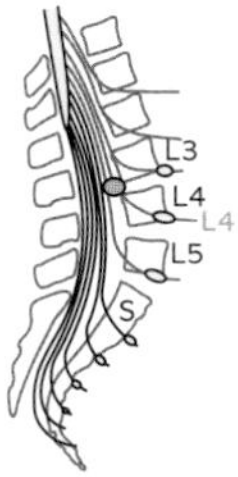 L3-4 disk; 4th lumbar nerve root | 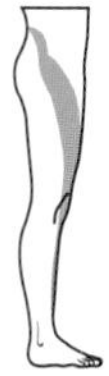 Lower back, hip, postero-lateral thigh, anterior leg | 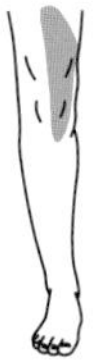 Anteromedial thigh and knee | Quadriceps | 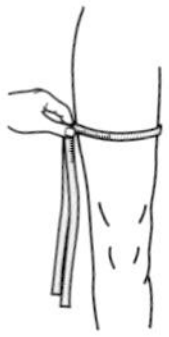 Quadriceps | 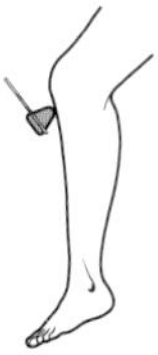 Knee jerk diminished |
| 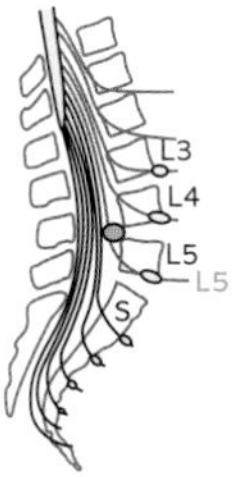 L4-5 disk; 5th lumbar nerve root | 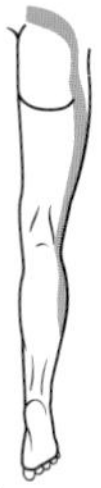 Over sacroiliac joint, hip, lateral thigh and leg | 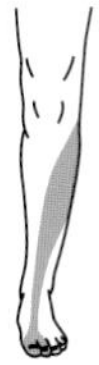 Lateral leg; first 3 toes | 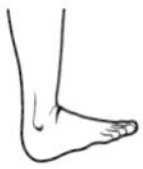 Dorsiflexion of great toe and foot; difficulty walking on heels; foot drop may occur | Minor | Changes uncommon in knee and ankle jerks, but internal hamstring reflex diminished or absent |
| 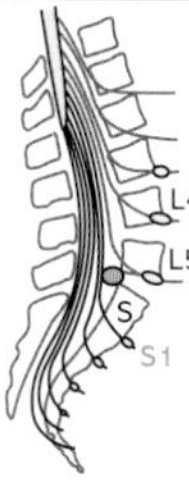 L5-S1 disk; 1st sacral nerve root | 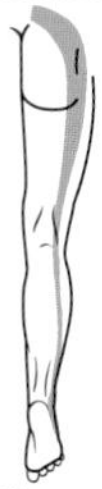 Over sacroiliac joint, hip, postero-lateral thigh and leg to heel | 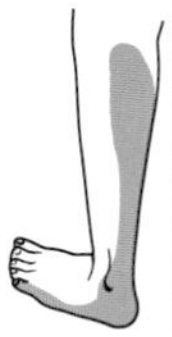 Back of calf; lateral heel, foot and toe | Plantar flexion of foot and great toe may be affected; difficulty walking on toes | 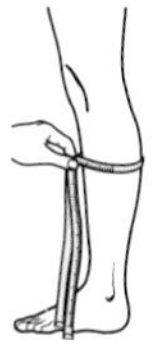 Gastrocnemius and soleus | 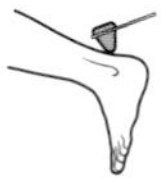 Ankle jerk diminished or absent |

**Figure 2.4** Clinical features of a herniated lumbar disk at L3–L4 (relatively rare), L4–L5 or L5–S1.

TABLE 2.3

**Examination pointers for assessment of spinal alignment**

- Where is the pain?
- Is the pain diffuse or focal?
- Is pain associated with a specific movement?
- Are there focal areas of tenderness and, if so, where are they located?
- Is the pain on a spinous process, an interspinous ligament or in the adjacent paraspinal muscles?
- Is the pain felt on deep probing over a facet joint area, or is it on the posterior iliac spine?
- Does flexion increase pain intensity or cause demonstrable muscle spasm (suggesting an annular strain or midline disk protrusion), and if so, by what degree of flexion?
- Does the pain lateralize during flexion (suggesting a possible disk herniation)?
- Does the pain lateralize during extension or side-bending?
- Does the pain radiate in a specific neural or radicular distribution, and if so, is this associated with sensory alterations, facet joint involvement, annular tears or disk rupture?

Diffuse pain is usually a function of pain severity. It can represent an individual's general low pain tolerance as in fibromyalgia, or it can be an indicator of ankylosing spondylitis or a possible fracture, infection or tumor.

## Palpation

Palpation of regions or foci of tenderness is helpful in establishing a basis for pain referral patterns, and may identify specific lesions, e.g. bursitis, or muscle trigger points and ligament and tendon insertion areas that may be amenable to local corticosteroid or local anesthetic injections. The identification of classic symmetrical trigger points and tender points is essential to the diagnosis of fibromyalgia (Figure 2.5).

The most commonly detected tender and trigger points associated with low back pain are shown in Figure 2.6 and are listed below in the

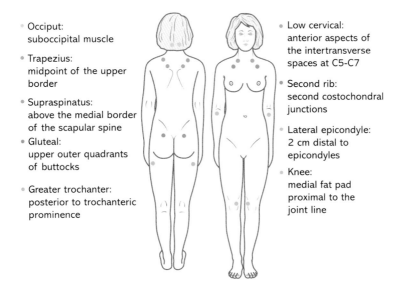

Occiput:
suboccipital muscle

Trapezius:
midpoint of the upper
border

Supraspinatus:
above the medial border
of the scapular spine

Gluteal:
upper outer quadrants
of buttocks

Greater trochanter:
posterior to trochanteric
prominence

Low cervical:
anterior aspects of
the intertransverse
spaces at C5-C7

Second rib:
second costochondral
junctions

Lateral epicondyle:
2 cm distal to
epicondyles

Knee:
medial fat pad
proximal to the
joint line

**Figure 2.5** Tender points that indicate the presence of fibromyalgia.

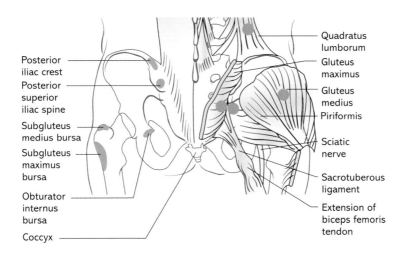

Posterior
iliac crest

Posterior
superior
iliac spine

Subgluteus
medius bursa

Subgluteus
maximus
bursa

Obturator
internus
bursa

Coccyx

Quadratus
lumborum

Gluteus
maximus

Gluteus
medius

Piriformis

Sciatic
nerve

Sacrotuberous
ligament

Extension of
biceps femoris
tendon

**Figure 2.6** The most common bone tender points and muscle trigger points to
consider on palpation of the lower back and pelvic regions

43

approximate order of the frequency of their manifestation in patients
with low back pain:
- the spinous process and interspinous ligaments of L4 or L5
- the sciatic outlet – piriformis trigger point
- the posterior superior iliac spine at the site of the iliolumbar ligament
  insertion, i.e. at the 'dimples of Venus'

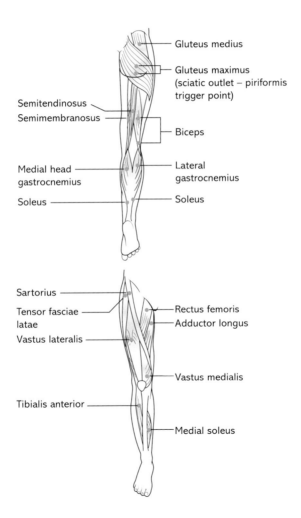

**Figure 2.7** Muscle tender points of the legs are focal areas of referred muscle
tenderness associated with disk disorders or hip or knee arthritis.

- the submaximus trochanteric bursa
- the facet joints at L4–L5–S1
- the posterior iliac crest
- the obturator internis bursa
- the quadratus lumborum trigger point
- the subgluteus medius bursa.

Muscle tender points of the legs are shown in Figure 2.7.

## The FABERE hip arthritis stretch

Hip arthritis, which mimics L2–L4 radiculopathy, is a commonly overlooked diagnosis in patients with low back pain and apparent sciatica, and the FABERE (Flexion, Abduction, External Rotation, Extension) hip motion test (Figure 2.8) should be an essential component of the back examination where this possibility exists.

Hip arthritis pain is referred to the thigh and often to the knee. Submaximus trochanteric bursitis is also commonly found and can be associated with referred 'pseudo-sciatica' in the lateral thigh. The L2–L3 lateral femoral cutaneous nerve distribution in the lateral thigh overlaps the area of pain referral from the submaximus trochanteric bursa. Submaximus trochanteric bursitis can sometimes produce

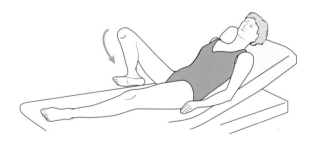

**Figure 2.8** The FABERE (Flexion, Abduction, External Rotation, Extension) hip arthritis stretch. If hip arthritis is suspected, the FABERE maneuver is done gradually to test for restricted and/or painful hip joint mobility.

dysesthesias in essentially the same lateral thigh region and can very occasionally refer pain into the groin.

- If when asked, or on the pain drawing, the patient indicates the location of pain in the proximal thigh and groin, there is a strong possibility that hip arthritis is the cause.
- Tenderness on palpation over the anterior hip capsule, in the absence of a hernia or inguinal adenopathy, is highly suggestive of hip joint arthritis.
- If the range of motion of the hip is restricted, and pain is elicited at the extremes of FABERE hip joint motion testing, hip arthritis is the probable culprit.

## Neurological testing

The sequence of testing neurological reflexes is arbitrary.

**The Romberg test** for peripheral neuropathy and balance can be performed at any time the patient is standing, or at the time gait or functional muscle tests are done. The patient is relaxed. Patient is asked to stand with his/her feet together and head erect. When stable, the patient is asked to close his/her eyes. The Romberg test is positive if the patient demonstrates increased unsteadiness with the eyes closed. This test when positive suggests the possibility of a number of neurological dysfunctions, from cerebral arteriosclerosis to peripheral neuropathies.

**The Babinski test** for upper motor neuron dysfunction can be done in conjunction with the ankle jerk reflex test, or when vibratory sensation is tested. The patient can be tested seated or supine without stockings. The plantar surface of the foot is then firmly stroked (utilizing a blunt object such as the handle of a reflex hammer). Normally the great toe will plantar flex. If dorsiflexion occurs, the plantar reflex is then demonstrating a positive Babinski – indicative of an upper motor neuron dysfunction. This also provides another opportunity to observe and possibly measure lower extremity atrophy and edema, and to note arthritic joint swelling and tenderness, as well as dermatologic disorders, scarring, contractures, varicosities, possible phlebitis, arterial pulse deficiencies and ischemia.

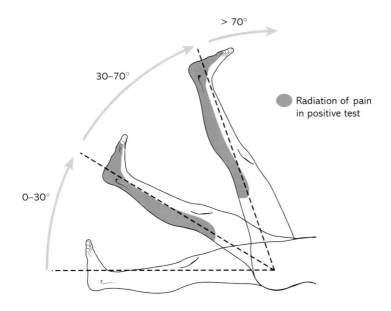

**Figure 2.9** The straight leg raise test for sciatic nerve impingement.

## Sciatic nerve impingement and hip joint testing

**The straight leg raise** is the classic test for sciatic nerve impingement
of the two lower nerve roots (Figure 2.9). This is performed with the
patient supine with the 'good' leg and knee extended on the examining
table. The symptomatic leg is then slowly raised while keeping the knee
extended: sciatic pain provoked at less than 30° is very suggestive.

*The crossed straight leg test.* An even stronger indicator of sciatic
nerve involvement, however, is obtained in the crossed straight leg test
if sciatic radiation in the opposite (involved) side occurs during straight
leg raising of the asymptomatic leg. It should be noted that when a
patient is recovering from a sciatic impingement, the angle of straight
leg raising required to provoke the sciatic pain increases. This is also
relevant to milder cases of sciatica, which may present initially with
unresponsive straight leg raising until the tested leg reaches 50–70°.
The following should be noted.

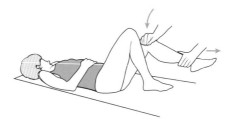

**Figure 2.10** The Lasègue test. Lasègue's sign: extension of the knee causes pain along the sciatic nerve.

- Tight hamstring muscles, when stretched, can cause pain to be referred to the thighs, thus greatly reducing the usefulness of the test.
- A straight leg raise test with the patient seated that does not provoke sciatic pain after the patient was strongly positive on the conventional supine straight leg raise test is considered to be an indicator of malingering or, perhaps more politely, gross exaggeration.

**The Lasègue test** also detects sciatic nerve impingements (Figure 2.10). It is most useful for patients who cannot lie fully supine because of their back pain. With the back on the table, the hips and knees are flexed so that the feet are placed flat on the table. The involved leg is supported and slowly extended to test for sciatic irritability. Although it is more difficult to measure the degree of leg raising, thereby making this test less precise, nonetheless it provides a useful alternative to the straight leg raise test for patients who could not otherwise be tested.

**The femoral nerve stretch test** is designed to detect nerve root irritability in the L2–L4 nerve roots (Figure 2.11). The patient is positioned prone with both legs extended (a pillow placed under the abdomen may make this less uncomfortable), and the affected hip is slowly extended with the knee slightly flexed. Pain and/or dysesthesias radiating down the front of the thigh is indicative of nerve root impingement. Like the crossed straight leg test, the crossed femoral nerve stretch test has enhanced specificity for nerve root impingement.

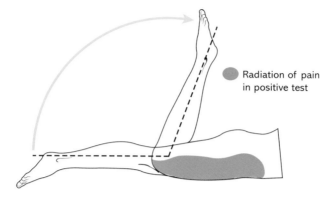

Radiation of pain
in positive test

Figure 2.11 The femoral nerve stretch test.

## Reflex and sensory distributions

The signs and symptoms associated with involvement of lumbosacral nerve roots are given in Figure 2.4. Sensory dermatomes are illustrated in Figure 2.12.

**Sensory nerves.** The sensory examination can be simply performed with a small brush to test light touch, and a pin for two-point discrimination (at 2–3 mm pin-point separations). A tuning fork is used to test vibratory sensation over bony prominences, e.g. the lateral malleolus or the proximal phalanx of the great toes, as a possible marker of associated peripheral neuropathy, most commonly diabetic neuropathy. The distribution of the sensory nerve and radicular patterns of impaired sensation are important in determining the nature and locations of the neural impairments. In those cases where the sensory distributions are unclear or absent, motor reflexes and/or muscle strength testing may prove more definitive, and electrodiagnostic testing may be a consideration (see page 59).

**Reflexes.** The key nerve roots that are usually tested first are:
- L2–L4 (most often L4) by the knee jerk (quadriceps) reflex
- L4–S1 (particularly the L5) by the medial hamstring (semimembranosus) tendon reflex
- L5–S2 (primarily S1) by the ankle jerk (gastrocnemius/soleus) reflex.

49

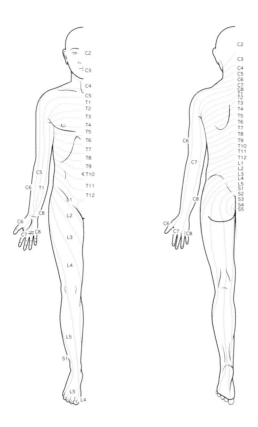

**Figure 2.12** Spinal sensory dermatomes.

A hypoactive medial hamstring (L5) reflex is sometimes the only positive confirmatory reflex finding. It can be elicited with the patient sitting or supine, with the knee flexed and relaxed. Digital pressure is placed firmly against the tendon posterior to the knee joint, and the tendon is then struck with the reflex hammer in a manner similar to that used to elicit a biceps brachialis reflex.

## Muscle testing

The aim of muscle testing is to note muscle atrophy and to assess:

- muscle function
- muscle strength.

An overall lower extremity and trunk strength and balance test can be quickly done, by simply asking the patient to sit and then rise. This gives a global overview of trunk and lower extremity muscle functioning, balance and coordination, and may identify areas of weakness needing more precise evaluation.

**Muscle atrophy**, if noted, can be bilaterally measured circumferentially at the widest region of the muscle.

**Functional muscle testing** is usually the quickest and easiest to perform unless the patient is in too great discomfort, in which case reliance must be placed on the manual muscle test (see below). The patient can be readily monitored for pain, imbalance, arthropathies and deformities while assessing possible weakness. The Romberg test (see above) can be the initial test, followed by observation of the gait (only a few steps in the examining room or preferably a walk in the hallway are required), noting any abnormalities such as scoliosis, foot drop or imbalance.

**Functional muscle strength.** After the Romberg and the gait tests, the patient should be asked to stand with both feet side by side and comfortably flat on the floor. Then they are asked to raise each forefoot and, if possible, walk a few steps bearing weight only on the heels – to test ankle and long toe extensors (tibialis anterior, extensor digitorum longus, peroneus muscles), L4–L5 and S1. The patient is then asked to stand on the toes of both feet. If this is successful, the feet are again placed flat on the floor, and the patient is asked to rise on the toes of first one foot and then the other, and then attempt to walk on the toes – to test foot and ankle stabilizers and toe and foot flexors (gastrocnemius/soleus, flexor digitorum), L4 and S1–S2. Finally, the patient is asked to attempt to do a deep knee-bend and arise – quadriceps, L2, L3, L4.

**Manual muscle testing.** The muscle groups tested functionally can also be evaluated by manual muscle tests, which are particularly valuable for patients who cannot perform the functional tests. They can also help to identify the weakened muscle more specifically.

With the patient seated or lying down to avoid pain, the muscles are tested by the examiner placing a hand over the distal area to be tested, e.g. the great toe for the long toe extensor, the metatarsophalangeal joints for the ankle dorsiflexors. The patient is asked to resist the examiner's pressure. Resistance is then scored 0–5 (Table 2.4). Subtle signs of unilateral weakness can be detected by asymmetry of responses, and malingering is suspected when responses are inconsistent on consecutive tests.

The muscle groups tested are a function of the patient's symptoms. Those most readily tested are:

- the toe extensors and flexors
- the ankle extensors and flexors
- the knee extensors and flexors
- the hip extensors and flexors.

Equivocal or conflicting findings of muscle weakness or dysfunction can be more precisely assessed by electrodiagnosis, and in particular by electromyography (see electrodiagnostic studies on page 59).

Manual muscle strength testing is at best a subjective evaluation, depending on the examiner's grading in conjunction with the patient's

TABLE 2.4

**Manual muscle test scoring**

|  | Score |  |
| --- | --- | --- |
| Normal | 5 | Full manual resistance of muscle group tested at end of range against gravity |
| Good | 4 | Detectable weakness at end of full range against gravity plus manual resistance |
| Fair | 3 | Ability to move through full range against gravity but unable to support added manual resistance |
| Poor | 2 | Ability to move through range with gravity eliminated |
| Trace | 1 | Minimal or no visible contraction |

Pain will nullify test grading
Source: Daniels L, Worthingham C. *Muscle Testing Techniques of Manual Examination*. Philadelphia: WB Saunders, 1986:2–5

cooperation. If performed consistently by the same examiner, however, the scores are reasonably reproducible, and are useful both diagnostically and prognostically, in terms of assessing patient progress.

---

### Clinical assessment – Key points

- 'Red flags' are a set of findings that suggest that back pain is non-discogenic and may be due to fracture, malignancy or infection.
- The VAS (visual analog scale) is a simple linear scale to measure pain intensity and response to therapy.
- The pain drawing provides a very simple way for the patient to indicate the region of the pain and often suggest etiology. A classic example indicates groin tenderness as a marker of probable hip joint rather than back-referred disorder.
- Ergonomic factors should be assessed, and this can often be readily done by observing the patient's conduct in the clinic and during examination.
- Palpation of key painful areas of the spine, facet joint areas, iliac crests, buttocks (sciatic outlet – piriformis region) and trochanteric bursae will often indicate the nature of the pain and/or significant areas of referred pain that may respond to therapy.
- The patient's gait and body motion can be observed in the clinic to detect sciatic scoliosis, short leg, hip, knee or foot arthritis or weakness and/or foot drop as markers of relevant pathology.

---

### Key references

Swezey RL, ed. Low back pain. *Phys Med Rehabil Clin N Am* 1998;9:309–523.

Wisneski RJ, Garfin SR, Rothman RH, Lutz GE. Lumbar disc disease. In: Herkowitz HN, Garfin SR, Balderston RA et al., eds. *Rothman–Simeone: The Spine*, 4th edn. Philadelphia: WB Saunders, 1999:613–79.

It is relatively easy to think of further tests that could be performed after an initial clinical diagnosis has been made, but it is important to decide which, if any, of these will increase our understanding of the patient's problem. As the cause of almost all low back pain disorders cannot be precisely characterized, some diagnostic limitations must be accepted. However, the physician may be under pressure from the patient or family to perform 'all the necessary tests', or from a medical insurer not to perform them, and may also feel under medicolegal pressure.

The main options for further investigations are:

- radiology
- electrodiagnostic studies
- laboratory studies.

## Radiology

Many patients over 40 years of age show some disk space narrowing and/or osteophytic spurs or spondylolisthesis on radiographs, and identifiable radiographic abnormalities are found in almost all individuals over 50 years old. In addition, disk bulges, protrusions, or extrusions at one or more vertebral levels have been identified by MRI in over 50% of asymptomatic subjects, and these are often perceived as the causal factor of their low back pain. In view of these statistics, and as pain cannot be assessed from a radiological scan of any type, it is worthwhile considering when, and whether if at all, the various radiological techniques are appropriate.

In geriatric patients, there are often many more abnormalities than necessary to explain the acute, subacute or chronic painful disorder. Further, when remission of symptoms occurs, in all likelihood the osseous abnormalities will remain unchanged, and even the soft-tissue disk-related lesions will still be present or little changed. This has been confirmed in several studies comparing a baseline MRI taken for a symptomatic disk derangement with a follow-up MRI.

**Radiography.** In a young and otherwise healthy patient who develops acute low back pain after bending and lifting or during vigorous sport activities, radiography or other radiological assessment serves only to reassure the anxious patient or family, and possibly establish a baseline for future comparisons, and there is little likelihood of discovering a significant abnormality. A minimum 4–6-week deferment of radiological testing to allow for the usual spontaneous improvement to occur is appropriate. At this time, recurrent low back pain or signs of spondylolisthesis should be the signal for greater long-term emphasis on ergonomic functioning.

In contrast, however, significant radiographic findings are highly likely in a patient with low back pain and/or sciatica and evidence of any of the 'red flags' (see Table 2.1 on page 33), or in a patient who has suffered a severe trauma capable of causing a fracture. Osteoporotic fractures can potentially occur in any part of the spine, though they are typically found in the thoracic and upper lumbar spine, and are less common in the lower lumbar vertebrae and rare in the cervical spine. Low back pain associated with osteoporosis and a lower lumbar fracture (L3–L5) is possibly tumor-related, though benign and malignant tumors may occur anywhere in the spine. Vertebral tumors can be confused with atraumatic or traumatic osteoporotic fractures (Figure 3.1), but are most likely in patients with night pain or in those whose pain is not relieved by rest. Bony lesions in these patients may be better characterized by CT.

If Reiter's syndrome or a related spondyloarthropathy is suspected, radiography of the pelvis will usually easily identify characteristic sacroiliitis and spinal longitudinal ligament ossifications (bamboo spine if severe). These sacroiliac lesions may be identified earlier, however, and monitored more easily during treatment, by MRI.

Flexion and extension view radiographs can very occasionally assist in assessing abnormal intervertebral motion and instability in cases of spondylolisthesis or scoliosis (Figure 3.2).

**Discography** consists of injecting a radiopaque substance under fluoroscopic guidance into the intradiscal space. Intradiscal contrast injections have been used as a diagnostic tool for disk-related

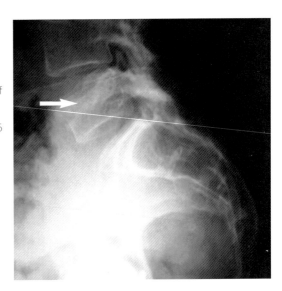

**Figure 3.1**
Osteoporotic fracture of
the 5th lumbar
vertebra, with the L4–5
disk compressing its
superior endplate and
underlying fragile
vertebral tissue.

pathologies for over 35 years, but the technique is associated with a
high rate of both false-positive and false-negative findings. In a geriatric
population and for patients with chronic pain, the specificity is only

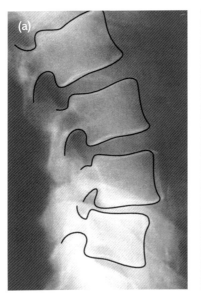
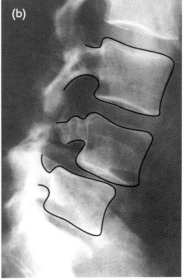

**Figure 3.2** Spondylolisthesis of L4 over L5, in association with disk degeneration,
is (a) partially ameliorated in extension and (b) accentuated in flexion.

about 20%. The ability of patients to localize a specific disk derangement by pain-provoking stimulations during discography, and to relate the provoked pain to their symptoms, is also unreliable.

**MRI.** Soft tissue abnormalities, disk protrusions, infections, cysts, tumors and facet joint arthritis are characterized better by MRI than by radiography, though the findings may still be poorly correlated with clinical findings. MRI is more sensitive than either radiography or CT in identifying abnormalities in patients with low back pain, and does not carry the risk of x-ray exposure, but it is more expensive and more likely to provide worrisome detail rather than useful information.

Disk abnormality descriptions are very important in patients with low back pain, but the nomenclature used to describe disk abnormalities is not standardized, and this can lead to misinterpretation and overinterpretation of the radiological reports. The descriptions given below represent a partial consensus of the terminology used.

*Disk degeneration* is associated with a reduction in disk height (Figure 3.3).

*Annular fissures* are a possible marker of clinically significant disk pathology. They can be located concentrically, transversely or radially. Nuclear material displacing annular fibers and stimulating in-growth of blood vessels and sensory nerves in the anulus may be a possible mechanism for ongoing discogenic pain.

*A generalized disk bulge* is a small circumferential overlap of the anulus over the vertebral end-plates, and may be associated with slight disk space narrowing. However, a finding of an abnormal disk bulge may be coincidental and can often lead to unnecessarily aggressive treatment.

*A disk protrusion* is an asymmetrically located focal protrusion that extends into the spinal canal, but maintains intact some of the outer annular fibers. Large protrusions and extrusions are often associated with hematoma formation and edema, and thereby have a favorable prognosis for spontaneous resolution.

*A disk extrusion* extends through the anulus and the posterior longitudinal ligament into the epidural space. It may remain partly attached to the outer anulus or be positioned fully in the epidural

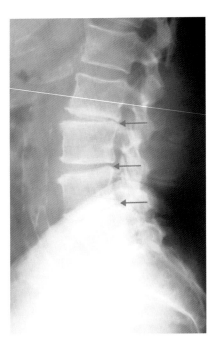

**Figure 3.3** Disk degeneration.

space, when it is termed a sequestration. Identification of a sequestration is important if surgery under microscopic visualization is undertaken.

The non-specific term 'disk herniation' is commonly used to describe protrusion or extrusion.

*Piriformis syndrome* consists of symptoms of sciatic radiculopathy associated with tenderness in the piriformis muscle region on deep palpation, and the absence of MRI or electrodiagnostic evidence of a disk protrusion. Because tenderness in the sciatic outlet / piriformis region is the most common pain referral manifestation of a lumbar strain with or without any nerve root impingement, the diagnosis of a piriformis syndrome is too often made. There are no negative consequences of this, however, unless unnecessary surgery is performed.

If an MRI of the lumbar spine shows no disk abnormalities, and if pathological enlargement of the piriformis muscle and displacement or entrapment is visualized by MRI of the sciatic nerve, therapy can be directed to relaxing and stretching the piriformis muscle or to the surgical release of the entrapped sciatic nerve tissue.

**Other radiological investigations.** Less commonly used radiological procedures include myelography and gadolinium-enhanced MRI.

*Myelography* utilizes a water-soluble contrast agent. It is used only occasionally, to assess the extent and precise location of a multi-level spinal stenosis.

*Gadolinium-enhanced MRI* can detect radiculitis, where there is a high correlation between marked nerve root enhancement and clinically relevant radiculopathy in patients with or without disk protrusions. It can also detect tumors and infections, and evaluate postoperative complications. However, mass effects on the thecal sack indicative of epidural fibrosis have been observed in more than 50% of patients tested in the immediate postoperative period and may persist for a year or more in successfully operated patients without any demonstrable, associated symptoms. With the possible exception of radiculopathy, these gadolinium-enhanced MRI scans reveal far more abnormalities than can be meaningfully interpreted.

**Interventional radiology** represents a new frontier in radiology. Several procedures are now utilized with increasing frequency by orthopedists, neurosurgeons and specialized intervention radiologists. These include selective nerve blocks, facet injections, epidural injections and percutaneous lumbar discectomies.

## Electrodiagnostic studies

When clinical testing for neurological defects is normal or equivocal, or when the radiological findings present too few or too many abnormalities to identify specifically the source of the neural abnormality, electrodiagnostic testing may add greater specificity. It can be particularly useful for distinguishing a unilateral distal peripheral neuropathy or entrapment from a disk-related nerve root impingement, or polyneuropathy from spinal stenosis. Although electrodiagnostic testing can confirm the presence of a nerve root lesion, it cannot indicate the precise level of the nerve root compression.

Electrodiagnostic testing consists of sensory nerve conduction studies – sensory evoked potentials (SEPs) and sensory F-wave latencies – and electromyography (EMG), which may be used singly or in combination.

*SEPs* measure sensory nerve conduction, which is most commonly affected by compression of nerve roots.

*Sensory F-wave latency* is mainly used to assess motor nerve functioning, but has slightly less sensitivity and no greater precision than EMG in determining nerve root compression levels. F-wave stimulation of the peroneal nerve is primarily conducted via the L5 and S1 nerve roots by the tibial nerve. The F-wave is generated by leg muscle stimulations transmitted via the nerve root to the anterior horn cells and then orthodromically to be recorded in the leg muscles.

**EMG** is the most sensitive electrodiagnostic method for detecting nerve root lesions, with precision reported as high as 78%. Nonetheless, the precision of EMG in one study of patients with clinical and radiographic (CT) findings of nerve root compression was as low as 20% when the EMG was correlated with surgical findings. It is also important to note that 'benign' fibrillations (the EMG marker for denervation) can be seen in normal subjects. Thus the interpretation of EMG abnormality is examiner-dependent, and the skill of the electrodiagnostician can be the crucial variable in interpretation of the test findings.

**Indications for electrodiagnostic studies.** Electrodiagnostic studies are not required for patients with low back pain of any severity if there is no subjective or objective evidence of nerve root impingement manifested by hypesthesia, asymmetric hypoactive reflexes, incontinence, sexual dysfunction, or muscle weakness.

Assuming that access to a competent electrodiagnostic consultant is available, electrodiagnostic studies are needed when:
- any of the above manifestations are present, but are not readily explained by the physical or radiological findings
- the patient cannot cooperate in the examination because of psychological or pharmacological (medication sedation) problems
- there is more than one apparent cause of the neurological findings (diabetic neuropathy, prior sciatica, traumatic peripheral neuropathy, spinal cord injury or tumor, myopathy, dystrophy or multiple sclerosis, among others).

> **Investigations – Key points**
>
> - Radiology: over age 40, disk degeneration and protrusions and osteophytes are common, and over age 50 almost universal.
> - In geriatric patients, radiographic evidence of spinal degeneration may be disregarded unless a tumor, osteoporotic fracture, infection or severe spinal stenosis is noted.
> - Geriatric radiographic abnormalities tend to persist after a patient goes into remission.
> - Discography is a relatively unreliable method of determining the locus of disk symptomatology, with numerous false positives.
> - When CT/MRI and the examination do not define the pathology, electromyography (EMG) may be helpful, but at best this has less than 80% accuracy in detecting a nerve root lesion.
> - Laboratory tests usually are not needed for acute low back pain unless 'red flags' are present or for patient monitoring to avoid potential hematological, hepatic or renal drug-related complications.

It should be remembered, however, that for most low back pain syndromes, a careful history and examination and radiological studies will provide the necessary information for starting appropriate conservative therapies, or for considering surgical intervention, even without electrodiagnostic testing.

## Laboratory testing

For the most part, with the exception of patients with 'red flags' (see Table 2.1 on page 33), laboratory testing for patients with low back pain disorders is of little value. Clearly, when malignancy is suspected, or osteoporotic fractures are identified, appropriate testing is warranted. However, the possibility that an HLA-B27 test and determination of erythrocyte sedimentation rate may help to confirm a suspected diagnosis of ankylosing spondylitis should be considered. Laboratory tests are most useful if medical complications, e.g. renal

61

and hepatic diseases, diabetes or infection, are suspected or have previously been confirmed. The usual indication for blood and urine laboratory testing is to monitor tolerance of pharmacological therapies and their potential side-effects.

**Key references**

Swezey RL, ed. Low back pain. *Phys Med Rehabil Clin N Am* 1998;9:309–523.

Tullberg T, Svanborg E, Isacsson J, Grane P. A preoperative and postoperative study of the accuracy and value of electrodiagnosis in patients with lumbosacral disk herniation. *Spine* 1993;18:837–42.

A broad spectrum of therapeutic options is available for the treatment of low back pain. Unfortunately, the efficacy of most, if not all, of the available remedies is not well established by research, and at least some of their effects can be attributed to a placebo effect.

In all phases of low back pain management, the patient must be given the responsibility and the tools to self-manage the disorder independently. In many acute lumbar strains nothing more than reassurance, cold compresses and analgesics may be required. In others this requires educational materials and careful instruction to the patient or a family member by the physician or therapist to ensure that all aspects of home treatments can be carried out as prescribed. The specific exercise at each phase of the progress toward normal activity, work and exercise should be monitored to ensure that it is properly performed and well tolerated.

## Principles of therapy

Therapeutic choices depend on both the chronicity and severity of the pain being treated. Chronicity is a measurable, time-dependent quantity (see Chapter 2, page 35), whereas severity can be highly subjective from both the patient's and the physician's perspective. A suggested grading system is shown in Table 4.1.

**Primary care.** The first 4 weeks of acute low back pain are generally managed by the primary care physician. For patients with acute, severe low back pain or an exacerbation of subacute or chronic pain and no 'red flags', the first priority is pain control, which may be necessary even before more definitive diagnostic procedures are undertaken. In addition to analgesic medication, RICE treatment is initiated, which consists of:

- Rest, ranging from limited activities to 1–2 days of bedrest, but with the patient encouraged to be ambulatory as much as possible
- Ice-cold compresses for 20 minutes per hour if needed
- Corset, or possibly a brace if previously used and properly fitted for comfort and support

TABLE 4.1

**Grading the severity of low back pain**

**Severe**
- The patient has any of the 'red flags' (see Table 2.1 on page 33)
- The patient is incapable of even minimal activity or unable to move without significant pain

**Moderate**
- Pain or sciatica is present most of the time
- Pain or sciatica prevents vigorous or prolonged customary daily activities

**Mild**
- Pain or sciatica is noticeable on straining, overuse or prolonged walking
- Pain or sciatica is noticeable on maintaining prolonged static postures such as bending in the garden, sitting in a movie or standing in one place

**Minimal**
- Pain or sciatica is only occasional and does not interfere with customary work or recreational activities

- Exercise, which may include gentle flexion or extension exercise to ease discomfort.

Prolonged bedrest should be avoided, as it has been shown to worsen outcome.

For a few patients with a painful radiculopathy not adequately relieved by RICE treatment, transcutaneous electric nerve stimulation (TENS) may provide some measure of pain control. This can help to minimize the need for higher doses of anti-inflammatory, corticosteroid or analgesic medications, and for epidural or nerve root injections and surgical procedures.

Depending on the patient's pain tolerance, the choice of medication becomes the next, and for severe pain the most urgent, therapeutic decision.

**Secondary care.** Specialist consultations are requested as needed during the subacute phase (5–12 weeks) of ongoing conservative management.

Treatments are allocated according to the severity of symptoms, and modified as dictated by the patient's response and/or compliance with the prescribed therapies. Treatments may include medication and rehabilitation therapies, with local trigger point, tender point, epidural and nerve root canal corticosteroid injections if indicated.

**Tertiary care.** If conservative therapies are judged to have failed, surgical procedures, if not otherwise contraindicated, are the appropriate treatment,

**Quaternary care.** For patients with chronic refractory pain or failed surgery, the treatment of choice is chronic pain management, for which specialized, multidisciplinary resources (typically including cognitive–behavioral management) are often required.

For patients with chronic, intractable, axial low back pain and/or leg pain, spinal cord stimulation using intraspinal canal implantable electrodes can provide pain relief that can be self-administered. Although it is not without risk, it may provide a reduced need for narcotics and, for some, a relatively narcotic-free pain control option.

## Medication

Although a few patients may request no medication, for almost all patients appropriate analgesic medication is the first priority. The US Agency for Health Care Policy and Research guidelines for medication use in low back pain are shown in Table 4.2.

**Analgesics.** The initial choice is usually analgesic medication available without prescription, including paracetamol, aspirin and a number of NSAIDs, e.g. ibuprofen and naproxen. These drugs in appropriate dosages are well tolerated, provided that known predisposing factors for side-effects are recognized and avoided, such as:

- liver disease and paracetamol
- gastrointestinal disorders, hypertension and renal disease and NSAIDs
- coagulation defects and aspirin
- geriatric vulnerability.

TABLE 4.2

US Agency for Health Care Policy and Research guidelines for the use of medications for low back pain

**Recommended medications**

- Acetaminophen (paracetamol)
- NSAIDs

**Medications considered optional**

- Muscle relaxants
- Opioids for less than 2 weeks

**Recommended against**

- Opioids for more than 2 weeks
- Phenylbutazone
- Oral steroids
- Colchicine
- Antidepressants

Analgesics offer relief particularly for patients who have pain and tenderness, but no major motion loss or neurological abnormality.

**Narcotics** are not uncommonly needed for a short-term pain control, and intermittently (on an as-required basis) for patients with subacute low back pain. The decision to administer narcotic analgesia to patients with chronic pain is more complex. The need for a moderate but effective dosage to control pain (rather than eliminate it) must be weighed against the risk of narcotic dependency, causing withdrawal symptoms if the drug is abruptly discontinued, and the possibility of addiction.

Tramadol, a non-scheduled, centrally acting analgesic for management of moderate to moderately severe pain, in combination with acetaminophen, has been investigated for the treatment of patients with chronic low back pain. These recent clinical studies suggest the combination tablet containing tramadol, 37.5 mg, and acetaminophen, 325 mg (Ultracet), is effective and safe as a 3-month treatment for chronic low back pain and provides improvement in quality of life measures related to physical and emotional functioning.

Narcotics vary in their analgesic effectiveness and tolerability for each patient. In general, codeine and dextropropoxyphene, with or without acetaminophen (paracetamol), aspirin or caffeine, tend to be less potent than oxycodone and acetaminophen, hydrocodone and acetaminophen, meperidine (pethidine), or morphine. These last two drugs are usually reserved for low back pain associated with severe trauma or intractable cancer. Long-acting, controlled-release analgesic formulations of narcotics, such as tramadol–acetaminophen (Ultracet) or a combination of oxycodone and acetaminophen, can offer better pain control and ultimately a lower total narcotic dose than as-required dosing, as peaks and troughs of pain (and hence of medication) are avoided.

**Anti-inflammatory agents.** Mechanical strains, probably because of an associated inflammatory response to tissue injury, may respond to the analgesic effects of both NSAIDs and short-term, high doses of corticosteroids.

*NSAIDs* are directed at primarily inflammatory disorders, e.g. ankylosing spondylitis. They appear to suppress inflammatory, cytokine-induced, chemically mediated aspects of lumbar discogenic spondylosis. Chemically induced pain with inflammation tends to be more persistent and less position-dependent than mechanically provoked pain. The inflammation associated with the irritated and inflamed annular tissue, adjacent nerve root and other neural structures, and the facet joints may be quite responsive to NSAIDs and to oral or injected corticosteroids.

The most common gastrointestinal side-effects of NSAIDs are:
• esophageal and gastrointestinal irritability
• peptic ulceration and perforation.
Gastrointestinal side-effects can be minimized by prescribing NSAIDs that inhibit cyclooxygenase 2 (Cox-2 NSAIDs) or by concomitant use of proton pump inhibitors or the prostaglandin analog misoprostol (which may itself cause side-effects). Other important side-effects of all NSAIDs include:

- hypertension
- fluid retention and edema
- congestive heart failure
- dermatitis
- exacerbation of renal and hepatic disorders.

*Oral corticosteroids.* High doses of oral corticosteroids are used when less aggressive treatments have failed, and every effort is being made to avoid surgery. Prednisone, 20–100 mg/day, or an equivalent dose of another corticosteroid, is given for approximately 5 days at a higher dose followed by up to several weeks at a lower dose, depending on the patient's response. High doses of corticosteroids, even for short durations, are not risk-free. In addition to drastic mood swings, susceptibility to infection, cardiovascular and gastrointestinal complications, avascular necrosis of a hip or other joint is an uncommon but potentially serious and uncontrollable complication.

In the UK, oral corticosteroids are rarely used in this setting, but epidural injection of saline and steroid (triamcinalone, 40 mg) is used.

**Psychiatric drugs.** Because psychological factors influence a patient's ability to cope with pain, effective pain relief should not only address the physical discomfort of low back pain, but also the psychopathology and pain-related psychological stress.

Psychiatric and skilled pain management assistance is often indicated for patients with intractable pain. Tricyclic antidepressants may be beneficial in patients with chronic pain and those suffering from fibromyalgia, particularly if night-time dosing minimizes daytime sedation while improving restful sleep. Selective serotonin reuptake inhibitors are not usually helpful in controlling low back pain, except in patients with both low back pain and unipolar or bipolar depressive mood disorders.

### Rehabilitation therapies

Rehabilitation therapies are directed at relieving pain and restoring function as far as possible. Therapeutic modalities and strategies are prescribed as needed at each stage of the low back pain syndrome, based on its severity and duration.

At various stages during rehabilitation, functional outcome can be assessed using one of five tests:

- the Sickness Impact Profile (SIP)
- the Roland–Morris Disability Scale (see page 37), derived from the SIP
- the Oswestry Low Back Pain Disability Questionnaire
- the visual analog scale (VAS)
- the Waddell Disability Index.

All of these can detect changes in the level of disability over time, though the Roland–Morris Disability Scale has been the most widely used.

**Back School.** The teaching aims of Back School are listed in Table 4.3, and are directed at providing patients with the basic tools to manage their back pain responsibly. Although a number of studies indicate a benefit of back schools, group education programs for both clinic patients and in industrial settings have not always proved effective. It has been argued that teaching patients strategies for self-care raises expectations and concerns, leading to inappropriate cure-seeking, and that low back pain should receive similar 'benign neglect' to the common cold. However, the healthcare system must take responsibility for providing patients with the basic knowledge required to function and exercise without aggravating their backs, or be guilty of neglect that is far from benign.

**Posture and ergonomics.** Bending, twisting and lifting are the most common activities that precipitate low back strain and pain.

TABLE 4.3

**Teaching aims of Back School**

- Appropriate exercises
- Proper use of medications
- Back-protective ergonomic functioning general principles
- Functioning at home, in the workplace, or while commuting

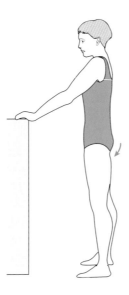

**Figure 4.1** The pelvic pinch (standing). The knees are comfortably relaxed and the buttocks squeezed gently together while simultaneously tightening the lower abdominal muscles.

Ergonomics are the key to minimizing stresses and strains and their consequent problems.

*Back first, back flat, back straight, back last.* 'Back first' emphasizes the need to plan ahead to avoid unnecessary back stressful activities. 'Back flat' reminds the patient to tighten the abdomen and gently squeeze the buttocks (pelvic pinch) to stabilize the back before initiating any new back movement (Figure 4.1). 'Back straight' is a reminder to stabilize the back and avoid bending, twisting and reaching. Finally, 'back last' is a message to use arms, legs, wheels and other aids, with the back the last thing put under any strain.

*Feet first and face it.* This is the key concept in avoiding twisting stress. The whole body should be turned from the feet upwards without twisting the torso before turning to perform any action, from reaching into a drawer to getting out of the car.

*Posture.* The 1-2-3–2 heads up posture is another important technique (Figure 4.2). The eye is aligned with an object straight in front (one finger), and then two fingers are used to push the chin back until a gentle stretch is felt at the back of the neck. Three fingers are used to press down on the vertex of the head while pushing the head up

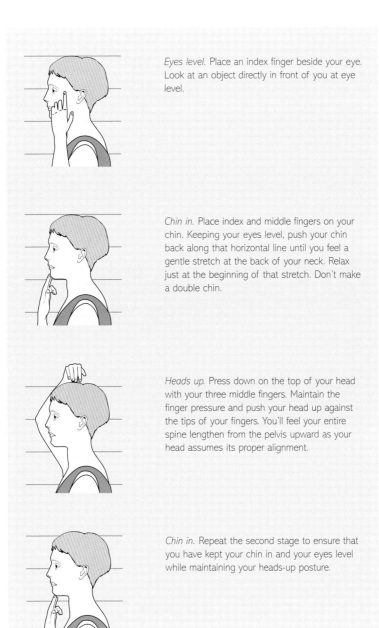

*Eyes level.* Place an index finger beside your eye. Look at an object directly in front of you at eye level.

*Chin in.* Place index and middle fingers on your chin. Keeping your eyes level, push your chin back along that horizontal line until you feel a gentle stretch at the back of your neck. Relax just at the beginning of that stretch. Don't make a double chin.

*Heads up.* Press down on the top of your head with your three middle fingers. Maintain the finger pressure and push your head up against the tips of your fingers. You'll feel your entire spine lengthen from the pelvis upward as your head assumes its proper alignment.

*Chin in.* Repeat the second stage to ensure that you have kept your chin in and your eyes level while maintaining your heads-up posture.

**Figure 4.2** The 1-2-3-2 heads-up posture. This sequence provides a reminder of how to balance the head over the torso.

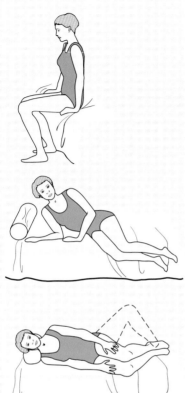

*Down*
Feel the edge of the bed with the backs of your legs. Place your more comfortable leg backward under the edge of the bed. Use your hands to help support you. Use your arms and hands to lift your buttocks and move back into a comfortable seated position on the bed.

Place both hands on the bed, on the side toward the head of the bed. Slide your hands toward the pillow to support your body as you gently swing your legs onto the bed. You should now be lying on your side.

Keeping your knees bent, place your hands on your thighs, do a pelvic pinch and roll onto your back, moving your shoulders, trunk and knees together as one unit – a 'log roll'. Adjust your legs one at a time for comfort.

*Up*
Lying on your back with your knees bent, do a pelvic pinch and hold. Holding the pelvic pinch, do a log roll to the side. Raise your shoulders by pushing off the bed with your hand and elbow; at the same time, gently swing both legs over the side of the bed. Use your arms and hands to help lift and slide your buttocks to the edge of the bed. Place one foot slightly in front of the other with your rear foot (your more comfortable foot) under the bed if possible. Keeping your buttocks tucked under (with a pelvic pinch) and your back straight, use your arms and legs to push up to a standing position.

**Figure 4.3** Lying down and getting up from bed.

against the pressure to lengthen the spine. Finally, the two-finger chin push to confirm head alignment is repeated. This posture method should be used sitting, standing or walking to balance the head over the torso, and can be combined with the pelvic pinch for perfect posture.

*Getting up and down.* Some of the maneuvers that are performed most often during the day can impose strains on the back and exacerbate pain. These include getting up and down from bed, chair, floor and squatting.

In order to get into bed, the patient should stand with the back of the legs in contact with the bed, and then sit while doing a firm but not forceful pelvic pinch (Figure 4.3). With both hands on the bed and leaning towards the head, the legs are gently swung on to the bed to achieve a side-lying position. Again while doing a pelvic pinch, the body is rolled as a unit (a log roll) on to the back and the legs adjusted one at a time for comfort. Getting out of bed involves the reverse. Similarly, sitting down requires the patient to stand with the back of the legs in contact with the chair. Then lower the buttocks on to the front of the chair while holding a pelvic pinch, and then move to the rear of the chair until the back is supported (Figure 4.4).

To reach the floor, the patient should be taught to first kneel on the stronger leg, using additional support such as a table or chair to maintain balance, while holding a pelvic pinch. The other knee is then put on the floor and the buttocks lowered on to the heels, keeping the back straight. Without twisting, the body is leaned to one side using both hands for support, the buttocks are shifted onto the floor and the body assumes a side-lying position, which can be modified by a log roll.

*Lifting.* Any objects should be lifted or put down by first squatting. Facing the object to be lifted with the stronger leg behind, the knees should be bent while holding a pelvic pinch and keeping the chin in (Figure 4.5). Standing from a squatting position is the reverse of these actions.

**Basic back protection.** Back pain can be reduced by appropriate planning.

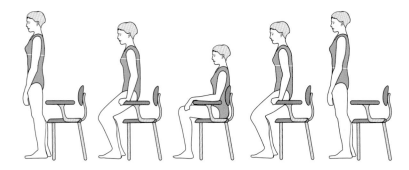

**Figure 4.4** Sitting down on, and standing up from, a chair. *Down:* feel the front of the chair with the backs of your legs. Place your more comfortable leg backward under the edge of the chair if possible. Do a pelvic pinch and, while holding it, bend your knees to lower yourself onto the front of the chair. Using your hands to support, move your buttocks to the rear of the chair until your back is supported. *Up:* using your hands on the arms or seat of the chair for support, move to the edge of the chair, keeping your back straight. Place one foot slightly in front of the other with your rear foot (your more comfortable foot) under the chair if possible. Keeping your buttocks tucked under (with a pelvic pinch) and your back straight, use your arms and legs to push up to a standing position.

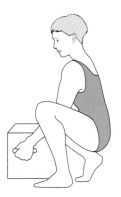

**Figure 4.5** To prepare for lifting, move close to the object or slide it close to your body; then squat or kneel before lifting. Bend your knees and keep your arms close to your body.

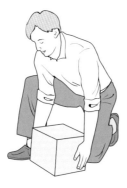

**Figure 4.6** A diagonal lift provides a good base of support when lifting heavy or awkward loads.

*Clothing* should be kept close, readily reached and easily donned. Reaching devices can be used when needed. Night and day clothes and underwear should be chosen for comfort and ease when donning, wearing and undressing. Stocking-donner devices can also help to minimize bending, twisting and pain.

Poorly fitted and loose shoes create balance and tripping problems. High heels and worn-out heels and soles can add to back discomfort by imposing postural strains. Pronated feet and foot and ankle arthritis can cause a back-stressing gait, and orthopedic shoes and orthotics should be considered. Elastic shoelaces and a long-handled shoe horn can minimize bending to don shoes and tie the laces.

Patients should avoid keeping their wallet in a back pocket, which can impose an awkward back straining posture while sitting for long periods of time. Bulky wallets should be stored in a jacket or coat pocket, or if this is not possible a seat cushion could be used to reduce the strain.

*Spectacles and hearing aids.* Straining to see or hear can impose awkward postures that make the patient vulnerable to back or neck strain, so the patient should be reminded to use spectacles and hearing aids whenever possible if these are normally required.

*Household organization.* The bathroom offers a number of challenges for back pain sufferers:
• a low toilet seat (a raised toilet seat appliance may be needed)

- difficulty standing in the shower or getting out of the bath (a grab bar or rail may be needed)
- bending to clean teeth and groom (fill a glass or cup full to avoid repeated bending, use a long and flexible straw, and place toilet articles on a box, a suitcase or an inverted drawer to minimize bending).

Household and work area equipment and furnishings should be rearranged for optimum accessibility and avoidance of bend and twist. Long handles, wheels, stools and ladders can also help.

**Beds.** The mattress should be firm, but not hard or lumpy. A plywood board can be placed beneath a sagging mattress for better support. The mattress should provide pressure equally to the head, shoulders and along the spine when lying supine or on the side. Prone positioning is best avoided, or modified by placing a pillow under the abdomen to relieve excessive lumbar lordosis and strain. Too soft a mattress permits prolonged resting in a suboptimal posture that promotes stiffness and pain. Soft polyurethane padding tends to compress over time.

The bed height should permit easy access. A chair, with the back adjacent to the bed, can provide support when getting in and out of bed. Adjustable electric beds can provide greater ease in bed positioning and for transferring in and out of bed.

The pillow should be soft enough to be comfortable when supine. It can then be folded to provide more thickness for head and neck support in the side-lying position. Pillows designed for neck support may also serve well.

**Seating.** The lumbar area of the chair should be firmly against the small of the back (Figure 4.7). For prolonged sitting, a small, self-inflating, adjustable pillow, or even a folded towel or sweater, placed between the back of the seat and the lumbar arch, can provide excellent seating tolerability. Portable seat and back supports are particularly helpful for car seating, and can be used in other settings where prolonged sitting is required. Soft-cushioned seating in chairs and couches should be avoided whenever possible.

The seat should allow the feet to be placed flat on the ground with the knees and thighs level. A footstool can be used for short legs. For

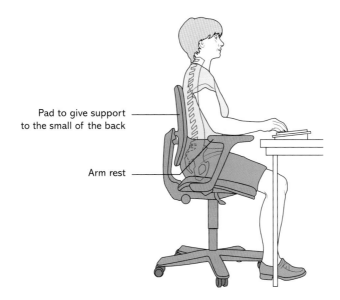

Pad to give support
to the small of the back

Arm rest

**Figure 4.7** A good seat for bad backs.

desk work, the legs should be able to slide under the desktop or any drawer underneath it. For working at a computer, a five-legged chair allows swiveling and working without twisting the back. Lighting for computer work should be glare-free and provide adequate visualization of the work.

*Standing.* Prolonged standing can impose a postural strain. When sitting is not an option, the use of small footstool, curb or box to bend one leg can permit more comfortable standing postures. For patients with spinal stenosis, leaning forward against a wall or a chair back can provide relief when it is not possible to sit. A cane (walking stick) with a folding-seat attachment is often helpful, as is a walker for the more infirm. These devices can permit more personal freedom for both walking and standing in line.

*Driving.* Disks are compressed by prolonged sitting and road vibrations, and truck and taxi drivers are very susceptible to low back pain. Any reaching for workloads, baggage, packages, small children, or to assist infirm parents makes the interdiscal tissues particularly vulnerable to strains.

Good car seat support is important for both drivers and passengers with back pain disorders. The car seat should be firm, or a firm seat and back supporting pad should be used. Bucket seats and slippery upholstered seating should be avoided. Seat adjustments should be made as needed. Long drives are best avoided. If they must be taken, patients should be advised to get out of the car and stretch every hour, and to sit so that the legs are not fully extended, with the knees slightly bent. On long journeys, lumbar and thoracic back supports, seat height and hip-to-pedal distances should be frequently adjusted. Particular care should be exercised when getting out of a car after prolonged sitting, especially if the seat arrangement is not optimal.

If possible when loading and unloading a car, packages should be placed in the passenger seat or the back seat close to the door. Objects should be placed as close to the rear of the trunk (boot) or the back of a sports utility vehicle as possible. The back ledge of the trunk can be used as a temporary holding or storage place while loading and unloading packages.

**Diet.** There is no specific diet for back pain. However, a balanced and nutritious diet with adequate fluids helps to avoid constipation or diarrhea and can minimize toilet-related back strain.

## Orthotics and assistive devices

*Corsets* can provide relief of acute and chronic back pain. Similar in function to a woven elastic bandage, they stabilize the spine and minimize strain. Simple cloth or elastic lumbosacral corsets that can be tightened in front with Velcro straps usually provide a measure of relief for acute low back pain. A dorsolumbar corset/brace can provide better support to the low thoracic and upper lumbar regions, but no corset can provide sufficient rigidity to actually prevent excessive lumbar movement under bending, lifting, reaching and twisting strains. Corsets and braces designed to be worn as back protection have not been shown to be protective. Corset fitting poses a considerable challenge for obese or pregnant patients.

After the first few weeks, a corset should be worn only at those times in the day when stressful back postures are likely. It is important to note that long-term use of a corset can weaken the paraspinal muscles and result in a weaker back that is more prone to develop further pain.

*Back braces*, which require customized fitting, are generally too cumbersome to don and wear for relief of back pain, except for patients with severe scoliotic or kyphotic deformities, or after operative fusions where a brace is needed to help maintain the spinal alignment.

*Walking sticks and leg braces.* Any leg condition that affects the gait should be addressed if possible in patients with severe, moderate or persistent back pain. Arthritic hip, knee, foot and ankle joints should, if possible, be treated in addition to the spinal disorder to minimize back stress related to pain-avoidance (antalgic) limping. Canes (walking sticks), crutches, leg braces and orthotics that facilitate a gait that is less antalgic, more balanced and less stressful to the spine should be used.

*Carrying aids.* Heavy purses, books, briefcases, shopping bags, tools or luggage should not be carried by hand if at all possible. Patients should use wheeled devices and ask for help, and shop in areas where one or other of these is available. Loads that must be carried should be divided into smaller packages whenever possible.

*Driving aids.* Using a wide-angle rear vision mirror can help to minimize painful twisting when driving, and especially when parking. If heavy packages need to be loaded or unloaded, patients should be encouraged to ask for help and to use wheeled carriers to move loads around.

## Therapeutic modalities

In addition to initial medication, and as back pain becomes less severe, local modalities, e.g. application of heat and/or cold, massage and stretching exercises, can be very effective in helping to soothe the pain. Whether these modalities add to the cure or simply add comfort during the natural healing process remains uncertain, largely because of a lack of controlled trials with adequate numbers of comparable cases. An exhaustive literature review reached the conclusions that:

- therapeutic exercises are beneficial for chronic, subacute and post-surgical low back pain

- continuation of normal activities is the only intervention with benefits for acute low back pain.

This review also indicated that, although heat/cold therapy, therapeutic ultrasound, massage and electric stimulation are possibly beneficial, definite evidence of their efficacy is lacking. However, it should be remembered that lack of proof does not necessarily mean lack of benefit, and provided that a treatment is safe, inexpensive and a comfort to the patient, it is worth offering. Back pain-relieving modalities followed by gentle exercise are almost always more useful than rest.

**Heat and cold.** After acute trauma or a muscular strain, application of a cold compress is usually the first modality to be used to control pain and to minimize bleeding and bruising. An ice-pack should not be applied for more than 20 minutes at a time, however, as this may very occasionally cause frost-bite or induce Raynaud's phenomenon. Cold compresses can very effectively relieve moderate-to-severe low back pain, and can also be soothing after a vigorous exercise or massage.

Heat, in the form of a shower or bath or as a dry or moist compress, is also a comforting modality which relaxes the muscles and facilitates any subsequent exercise, therapeutic or recreational. Heating an acutely traumatized area, however, can increase local bleeding and swelling. Prolonged heating with an electric heating pad, as may happen if the patient falls asleep, can cause a burn, and an alarm should be set for no more than 30 minutes.

**Ultrasound.** Application of ultrasound produces a deep heating effect. It is widely used for treatment of a variety of musculoskeletal disorders, including low back pain. Despite the lack of objective evidence of its efficacy, anecdotal experiences of patients and therapists suggest the opposite. Ultrasound is safe and may be helpful, and is worth trying.

**Diathermy.** Diathermy was once universally accepted as the state-of-the-art penetrating heat modality for almost all painful musculoskeletal disorders, but it has not stood the test of time. It has not been shown to have any advantage over other heating modalities that can be readily self-administered at home, and it requires special equipment and the cost of the therapist to administer it. Diathermy is no longer so widely employed.

**Traction.** Vertebral axial decompression of the lumbar disks by continuous motorized axial traction has been correlated with the extent of the traction force, but most studies have been unable to show significant improvement in clinical symptoms. The important exception may be spinal stenosis, in which horizontal traction applied for 30 minutes once or twice weekly has been reported to improve or stabilize symptoms of neurogenic claudication. Most patients with spinal stenosis report subjective benefits with lessening of overall discomfort and some increase in walking and standing tolerance after treatment with lumbar traction.

**TENS** (transcutaneous electrical nerve stimulation) is one of the few therapeutic modalities subjected to a serious attempt at double-blinded study. It was not possible to fully control for all confounding factors, and the outcome did not support a benefit for TENS treatment in chronic low back pain.

TENS has been shown to help relieve painful radiculopathies, however, and can offer a practical, non-pharmacological, patient-controlled therapeutic option. It can quickly be determined during an outpatient therapy visit whether TENS can provide adequate relief, in which case the patient can use it at home.

**Massage.** Most massage consists of gentle-to-firm muscle kneading movements which are usually soothing and relaxing, provided that excessive pressure or inappropriate attempts at manipulation are avoided. Massage can be administered as an overall body relaxation method, or specifically to the low back for pain relief.

*Acupressure* is a form of deep focal massage over specific acupuncture points that are considered relevant to relieving back pain and/or sciatic pain. The acupuncture and acupressure points are not uniformly used, and the benefits are not established.

*Rolfing* is a hybrid of massage and manipulation or mobilization that is used for myofascial pain syndromes. In back pain, the objective is to achieve a more vertical pelvic postural alignment by applying deep, firm pressure and vigorous kneading of the pelvic and lumbar musculature. Rolfing is often too painful, even in the hands of a trained Rolfing therapist, but some patients perceive a benefit.

**Manipulation.** Manipulation therapy administered by a skilled physician, osteopath, chiropractor or therapist can often expedite pain control during the first few weeks of an acute low back pain episode, as well during recurrences of a subacute or a chronic low back pain disorder. The objective is to release and realign impinged tissues (facet joint, intradiscal or sacroiliac joint, and/or adjacent neural structures), though the precise localization of any realignment has not yet been convincingly demonstrated. After 4 weeks, continued manipulations to achieve realignments of the spine for pain relief show little therapeutic efficacy, though up to that time chiropractic manipulation has been reported to have an advantage over McKenzie exercises (see page 84) or patient education. No long-term advantage, in terms of return to work and other functional or recreational activity, can be attributed to manipulation, and the patient may become dependent on manipulation for relief rather than learning self-administered therapeutic exercises or back-protective ergonomics.

Possible complications of manipulation, which are seldom reported, include death, paraplegia, and failure to diagnose accurately relevant coexisting medical disorders. Vigorous, abrupt spinal manipulation in the presence of a protruded disk and/or sciatic nerve root impingement risks further rupture of the anulus, disk extrusions and nerve root damage. Vigorous manipulation of an osteoporotic spine can also cause a fracture.

**Acupuncture** is another non-pharmacological and non-surgical therapy that may provide a measure of relief for acute, subacute and chronic low back pain patients, particularly for those who do not tolerate medication. Acupuncturists often also use a variety of herbal and topical remedies in addition to acupressure massage. Six treatments over a 2-week period are usually sufficient to determine if acupuncture can provide any pain control for an individual patient.

As with all low back pain therapies, however, there are both strong advocates and disappointed consumers of acupuncture treatment.

## Therapeutic exercises

From the standpoint of treating back pain, there are several levels of exercises. For the patient in pain, those exercises that can offer some relief and progressively restore, or at least maintain, function are therapeutic. In the absence of significant pain, exercises for posture correction, or overall stretching and conditioning, or any form of recreational exercise also have therapeutic value, but are not part of the back pain relief treatment per se.

For aerobic conditioning during the period of recovery from back pain, swimming is usually better tolerated than bicycling (with the seat-to-pedal distance adjusted to avoid spinal twisting while pedaling), which is better than jogging, which is better than rowing. Back-protected exercise activities should always be encouraged, not only for the back but also for cardiovascular and psychological reasons, as far as they are tolerated, though it must be remembered that well-intended conditioning exercises used by therapists and trainers for younger patients may prove disastrous for a geriatric back pain patient.

**Williams flexion exercises** have for many years been the gold standard of exercises for low back pain patients. They consist of six exercises designed to stretch the low back and the hamstring muscles, the ileolumbar ligament and the fascia lata, and to strengthen the abdominal and gluteal and quadriceps muscles. These exercises are performed progressively and as tolerated during convalescence. For most low back pain patients, they remain a good, basic conditioning exercise program.

The role of the abdominal muscles in providing back support during lifting activities is still controversial, and for many patients attempting to do a sit-up exercise can be painfully difficult. The use of a simple, supine isometric exercise, with the thighs vertically placed and the hands pushing against anterior aspect of the knees, provides an abdominal strengthening exercise that is usually well tolerated. This exercise also eliminates the risk of vigorous sit-ups that have been shown to provoke osteoporotic fractures, as well as potentially aggravate low back pain.

**McKenzie back extension exercises.** The McKenzie system for examining and treating low back pain disorders draws on the patient's history, a postural assessment, and active and passive movement tests to identify the lumbar derangement. The treatment is designed to 'centralize' a disk protrusion back into the nucleus pulposus. The McKenzie exercises consist of six graduated postures starting with prone lying and progressing to prone extension, and then standing hyperextension stretches. These postures are held for 10–15 seconds to achieve maximal tolerable restoration of lumbar extension.

When the back pain is accompanied by lateral deviation or shift of the torso, rather than just limited extension, this sciatic scoliosis is presumed to be due to either a protruding disk wedging and tilting the vertebrae, and hence the torso, mechanically, or to a pain-avoidance mechanism. Although trained therapists using the McKenzie protocol have not shown consistency in determining the presence, absence or direction of sciatic scoliosis, shift correction and centralization are often effective in relieving the associated pain.

Shift correction and centralization is a slow, steady horizontal squeezing of the torso over the pelvis. The rationale is to gradually return the protruding nuclear material to a more central disk location. The shift-correcting maneuver is performed to the extent tolerated and then taught to the patient to continue self-administration as needed to minimize the shift. After shift correction, the patient performs the back extension exercises which are intended to help maintain the centralized disk.

**Lumbar stabilization exercises** are a group of exercises designed to strengthen the abdominal, lumbar, gluteal, thigh and lower extremity muscles to maintain trunk alignment and back protection during daily activities. The use of the trunk muscles to maintain postural alignment helps to avoid stooping, twisting and consequent lumbosacral strain. The key to the stabilization approach is teaching awareness of an optimal, balanced, neutral spinal alignment, which is achieved by tilting the pelvis back and forth until a comfortable, balanced, pain-free mid-position is achieved. The patient then uses this posture during daily activities, for pain relief and to avoid twisting and bending stresses to the spine.

**Hamstring stretch.** Tight hamstring muscles restrict trunk flexion movements when standing and impose a much earlier stress on the lumbar spine. Stretching tightened hamstring muscles can be an important back-protective exercise in addition to lumbar, hip and thigh stretching.

**Alternative exercise techniques** offer a variety of ways to stretch, relax, contemplate and meditate. They can also provide, depending on individual views regarding the more conventional approaches to exercise, a mechanism for body stretching and strengthening that is enjoyable and hence will be more consistently performed.

Yoga is probably the most commonly used alternative posture and stretching exercise regimen. Others include the Alexander technique of posture training, the Mensendieck exercise and education program, the Feldenkrais method and the Pilates method. All these approaches should be well supervised, to ensure that they do not exacerbate back or other pain.

**Back-reconditioning exercises** form the core of the Swezey Institute Arthritis and Back Pain Center's treatment program for low back pain. They are graded depending on the level of pain, and the patient is cautioned to stop if any of them cause pain. Sample programs for patients with moderate pain or mild pain are given in Tables 4.4 and 4.5, and Figures 4.8–4.24. The patients work towards performing these exercises twice daily, and then (those with moderate back pain initially) progressing to exercises for mild back pain and finally to maintenance exercises. Once the patient has reached a level of back conditioning suitable for his/her normal daily activities, a once-daily maintenance exercise program can be started (Table 4.6 on page 102). Other forms of back-reconditioning exercises, such as core stability

TABLE 4.4

**Sample program of back-reconditioning exercises\* for patients with moderate low back pain**

- Double knee to chest
- Wall slide 30° angle
- Supine single straight leg raise
- Supine hamstring stretch
- Beginning pelvic rotation
- Partial sit-up (abdominal isometric)

\*See the list on page 8 to find each exercise

TABLE 4.5

**Sample program of back-reconditioning exercises\* for patients with mild low back pain**

- Crossed hip rotator
- Advanced pelvic rotation
- Supine hamstring stretch (opposite leg straight)
- Calf stretch (standing)
- Wall slide repetitions
- Cat back
- Quadruped (hands and knees) single arm raise
- Quadruped single leg raise
- Quadruped contralateral arm and leg raise

\*See the list on page 8 to find each exercise

exercises, can also be useful.

Another useful set of exercises is the 5-Minute Back Saver program. This program is designed to gradually warm the muscles so that they can be more easily stretched. The exercises are performed in the morning before breakfast, and can also be used to warm up and cool down before and after athletic activity. The program is described on pages 115–122.

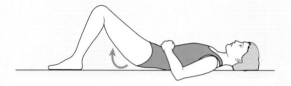

Lie on your back on a firm flat surface or on the floor (if you can get up again easily). Bend your knees and rest your feet flat on the surface. (A small pillow may be used under your head for comfort.) Place your hands on your abdomen, with your little fingers touching the top of your pelvis.

Squeeze your buttocks tightly together (imagine holding a coin between the buttocks). This flattens the back and initiates the pelvic tilt. Now tighten the abdominal muscles to complete the pelvic tilt. Hold this tilted position. *Do not hold your breath.* Count out loud from 1001 to 1006. Relax.

Repeat three to five times, once or twice hourly during the day when in bed, and at least twice daily during convalescence.

**Figure 4.8** Pelvic tilt. This exercise is the basis for all back conditioning and back protection postures. (The pelvic pinch, Figure 4.1, is a milder version.) It serves to relieve discomfort, stretch the low back (lumbosacral spine) and to begin to strengthen the abdominal and buttock (gluteal) muscles.

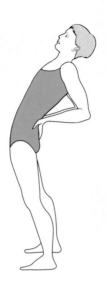

Stand in a straight-back posture with your feet a shoulder's width apart. Place your hands at waist level on each side of your back. Allow your thumbs to wrap around to the front and your fingers to lie over your low back. Keeping your knees straight and maintaining a chin-tucked position, relax your back and bend back at the waist In a steady, controlled manner; then return to the straight-back posture position. *Do not bend forward past the straight-back posture.* Say 'Pressure on; pressure off' as you repeat the movement.

Repeat ten times, once or twice hourly for pain relief, and five to ten times before, during and after strenuous or sustained activities or before and after your regular exercises.

*Caution:* Stop the exercise if pain increases in your legs or buttocks.

**Figure 4.9** Back bend, standing. It is now recognized that many patients will benefit from a slow repetitive back bend if it can be done without pinching the sciatic nerve or straining the small facet joints in the lower back. The concept is that leaning back squeezes bulging disk tissue forward. This can relieve pain and help prevent recurrences for patients suffering mild to moderate pain if done before and after strenuous or prolonged exercise or activity, or prolonged inactivity.

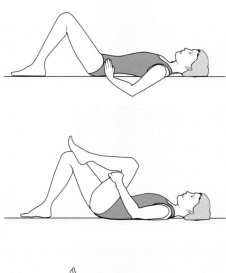

Lie on your back on the floor or another firm flat surface. Bend your knees, and rest your feet flat on the floor. (A small pillow may be used under your head for comfort.) Do a pelvic pinch and bend your knees.

Keeping your knees bent, slowly raise the leg that is on your more painful side.

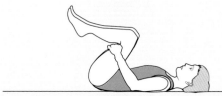

Then raise your opposite leg to join it. Release the pelvic pinch.

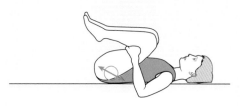

Grasp just behind your knees with both hands. Pull your knees gradually towards your chest until you feel a mild stretch in your lower back or at the back of your hip. Hold and count out loud: 1001, 1002, 1003. Breathe normally. Relax.

**Figure 4.10** Double knee to chest. This stretches the low back (lumbosacral) and buttock (gluteal) muscles.

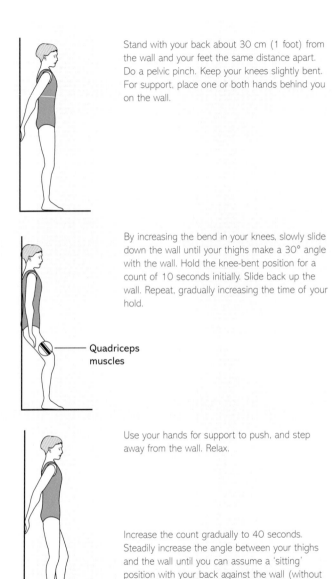

Stand with your back about 30 cm (1 foot) from the wall and your feet the same distance apart. Do a pelvic pinch. Keep your knees slightly bent. For support, place one or both hands behind you on the wall.

By increasing the bend in your knees, slowly slide down the wall until your thighs make a 30° angle with the wall. Hold the knee-bent position for a count of 10 seconds initially. Slide back up the wall. Repeat, gradually increasing the time of your hold.

Quadriceps muscles

Use your hands for support to push, and step away from the wall. Relax.

Increase the count gradually to 40 seconds. Steadily increase the angle between your thighs and the wall until you can assume a 'sitting' position with your back against the wall (without a seat) and hold it for 40 seconds. Do this exercise twice daily.

**Figure 4.11** Wall slide 30° angle. This helps to strengthen the quadriceps muscles in the thigh, and the buttock (gluteal) muscles, to improve control when squatting, sitting down and getting up from chairs.

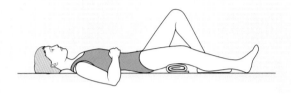

Lie on your back with both knees bent and your feet flat on the floor or other firm flat surface. Place a rolled towel or pillow under your right thigh just above the back of your knee. Keep your arms at your sides or on your stomach.

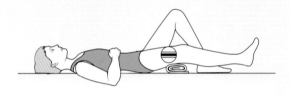

Do a pelvic pinch. Straighten your right leg. Keep your left leg bent. Press the back of your right thigh down into the towel or pillow as firmly as possible, and pull your right kneecap towards your thigh to tighten the quadriceps muscles. Do not arch your back. Try to increase your effort with every count as you hold and count out loud: Push 1, Push 2, Push 3, Push 4, Push 5, Push 6. Relax and bend your right leg. Place your foot flat on the floor.

Repeat the exercise with a towel or pillow under your left thigh, pressing the left thigh firmly into the towel or pillow. Repeat two times, twice daily until you are on a maintenance program.

**Figure 4.12** Quadriceps strengthener (single straight leg raise). This can be substituted for the wall slide (Figure 4.11) to help strengthen the quadriceps muscles when standing is difficult or painful because of foot, ankle, knee or hip problems.

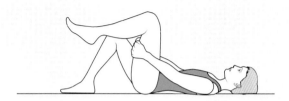

Lie down with your knees bent. Do a pelvic pinch. Bring your left knee half way to your chest. Keeping your neck and shoulders relaxed (to avoid neck strain), grasp your left thigh with both hands.

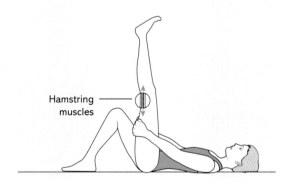

Relax the pelvic pinch. slowly straighten your left knee until you feel a stretch at the back of your knee. Keep your left foot relaxed. Hold and count out loud from 1001 to 1006. *Do not hold your breath*. Relax. Bend your left knee and return your foot to the starting position.

Repeat the exercise for your right leg. Repeat for each leg three to five times, twice daily until you are on a maintenance program.

**Figure 4.13** Supine hamstring stretch. This makes it easier to bend at the hips and avoid bending at the waist. (The low back is right on your beltline.)

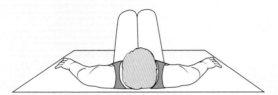

Lie on your back on the floor or other firm flat surface with both knees bent. Do a pelvic pinch. Place both hands at your sides with your palms down and about 50 cm (20 inches) away from your hips.

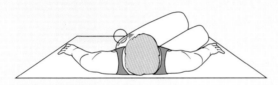

Moving both knees together, slowly rotate your hips to your right side as far as you can. You should feel a gentle stretch. Hold and count aloud from 1001 to 1006. Relax. Return to the starting position with both knees bent.

Repeat to the right side. Repeat for each side three to five times, twice daily (or once or twice each hour if it helps to relieve your back or buttock pain). Do the exercise once daily when on a maintenance program.

**Figure 4.14** Beginning pelvic rotation. This exercise can help to relieve pain on one side of your lower back or buttocks.

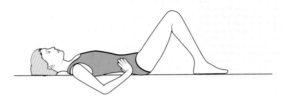

Lie on your back on the floor or another firm flat surface.
Bend your knees, and rest your feet flat on the floor. (A
small pillow may be used under your head for comfort.) Do
a pelvic pinch. If possible, hold the pinch throughout the
exercise.

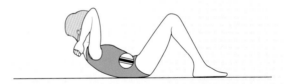

Grasp your hands at the base of your skull so that your *neck
is supported* by your hands. Keep your *chin tucked in*, and
use your abdominal muscles to slowly raise your head and
shoulders until your shoulder blades no longer touch the
floor. *Do not use your hands or neck to lift your shoulders.*
Hold and count out loud from 1001 to 1040 if possible. *Do
not hold your breath.* Return slowly to the starting position.
Relax.

Repeat one time, twice daily.

**Figure 4.15** Partial sit-up (abdominal isometric). This rather strenuous exercise
strengthens and tightens the abdominal muscles, which will decrease stress on
the low back. If neck or leg pain occurs, the knee push with chair exercise
(Figure 4.16) can be substituted.

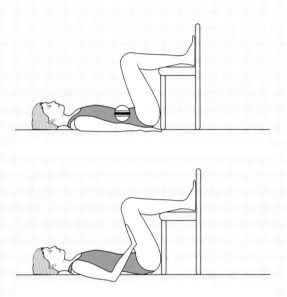

Lie on your back with your knees bent and your feet below a chair. Do a pelvic pinch. Slowly place the leg of your most painful side on the seat of the chair. Do the same with your opposite leg.

Keeping your upper arms flat on the floor and your elbows slightly bent, place your hands on your thighs. Do a forceful pelvic pinch as you push with your hands against your thighs. Resist the hand pressure with your thighs. Hold position and count out loud: 'Push 1, Push 2, Push 3, Push 4, Push 5, Push 6'. *Do not hold your breath.* Try to push harder with each count. Relax.

Slowly return your foot on the most painful side, and then your opposite foot, to the starting position.

Repeat ten times, twice per day; or hold for a count of 40, twice per day.

**Figure 4.16** Knee push with chair. This exercise can be substituted for the partial sit-up (Figure 4.15) when neck or leg pain is a problem.

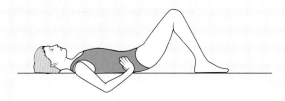

Lie on your back with both knees bent and your feet flat on the floor or other firm flat surface. Do a pelvic pinch and hold it.

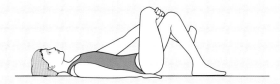

Cross your right leg over your left knee. Bring your right knee up toward your chest. Place your left hand around your right knee. Relax your pelvic pinch.

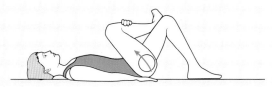

Gently pull your right knee toward your left shoulder with your left hand until you feel a slight stretch in your outer thigh and buttock. Hold this mild stretch and count out loud from 1001 to 1006. Relax, do a pelvic pinch and return to the starting position.

**Figure 4.17** Crossed hip rotator stretch. This good for stretching the thigh–buttock muscles and may help to prevent a strain when unavoidably twisting the low back. However, it can cause pain in the thigh, *so do it only if it feels good*. A slight change in the position of the upper leg may help to relieve discomfort.

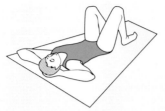

Lie on your back with both knees bent and your feet flat on the floor or other firm flat surface. Clasp your hands behind your head.

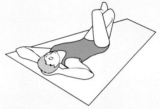

Cross your right leg over your left leg; place your right foot on the outside of your left leg, just below the knee. Do a pelvic pinch.

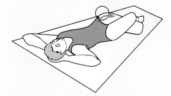

Keeping your upper back and shoulders stationary, use your right foot to steadily push your left knee toward the floor on your right side. You should feel a stretch in your left lower back or outer thigh as you try to touch your left knee to the floor. Hold the stretch for a count from 1001 to 1006. Return to the starting position. Relax.

Repeat the exercise with left and right reversed. Repeat three to five times for each side, twice daily, and once daily on your maintenance program.

**Figure 4.18** Advanced pelvic rotation. This exercise stretches the muscles that turn the low back and hips (external rotators). (It is also a good pre-athletic warm-up stretch.) It is not unusual to get a cracking sound in your back when you do this one, because the small facet joints can be momentarily separated (gapped). The crack is neither good nor bad, but the stretch often feels good and helps to restore mobility to the spine.

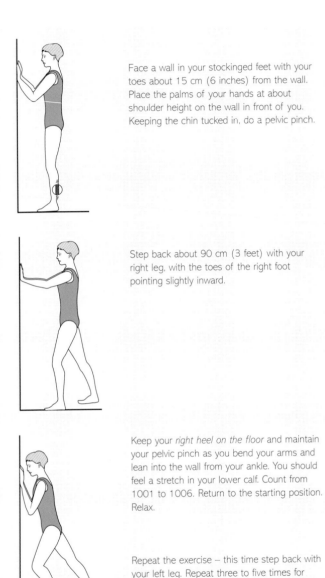

Face a wall in your stockinged feet with your toes about 15 cm (6 inches) from the wall. Place the palms of your hands at about shoulder height on the wall in front of you. Keeping the chin tucked in, do a pelvic pinch.

Step back about 90 cm (3 feet) with your right leg, with the toes of the right foot pointing slightly inward.

Keep your *right heel on the floor* and maintain your pelvic pinch as you bend your arms and lean into the wall from your ankle. You should feel a stretch in your lower calf. Count from 1001 to 1006. Return to the starting position. Relax.

Repeat the exercise – this time step back with your left leg. Repeat three to five times for each leg, twice daily, and once daily on your maintenance program.

**Figure 4.19** Calf stretch (standing). This exercise stretches the calf muscles and heel cords (Achilles tendons) so that, when walking or squatting, the leg and foot work properly and cramp is less likely. When tight, these muscles and tendons can pull the knee back, pull on the hamstrings and strain the back.

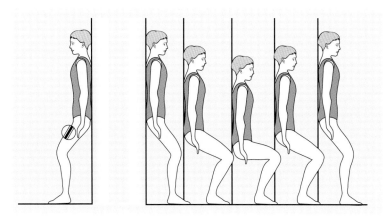

**Figure 4.20** Wall slide repetitions. This exercise is a good way to relieve back strain after prolonged sitting or standing. It conditions the leg muscles, especially the quadriceps in the thighs, for ease in squatting or arising. The procedure is as for Figure 4.11 except that you slide down until your thighs are perpendicular to the wall, then slide up again and repeat the sliding up and down three to five times as rapidly as possible. If needed, place a chair in front of you for balance. Repeat twice daily.

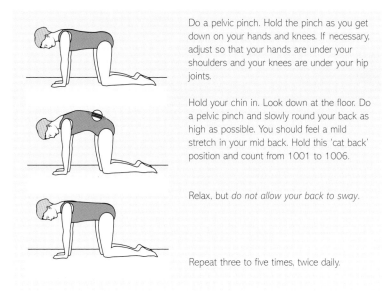

Do a pelvic pinch. Hold the pinch as you get down on your hands and knees. If necessary, adjust so that your hands are under your shoulders and your knees are under your hip joints.

Hold your chin in. Look down at the floor. Do a pelvic pinch and slowly round your back as high as possible. You should feel a mild stretch in your mid back. Hold this 'cat back' position and count from 1001 to 1006.

Relax, but *do not allow your back to sway*.

Repeat three to five times, twice daily.

**Figure 4.21** Quadruped (on hands and knees) cat back. This exercise helps to limber up the lower back.

99

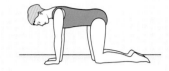

Do a pelvic pinch. Hold the pinch as you get down on your hands and knees. If necessary, adjust so that your hands are under your shoulders and your knees are under your hip joints.

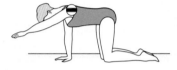

Hold your chin in. Look down at the floor. Do a pelvic pinch and raise your left arm about 30 cm (1 foot) off the floor. (Keep the arm below shoulder height.) Hold and count out loud from 1001 to 1006.

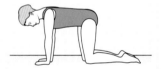

Put your arm down. Relax, but *do not allow your back to sway*. Repeat the exercise using your right arm as instructed.

*Sequence.* Initially, try this exercise holding once for a count of six. If you have done this for 2 days without any problems, repeat it twice for a count of six, and then do that twice daily for a week. After 1 week, add the exercise shown in Figure 4.23 and proceed in the same manner. Wait 2 more weeks before adding the exercise shown in Figure 4.24, and do so only if all is going well. In that exercise, you can gradually increase to a count of twenty in each position, repeating them twice and doing the exercise twice daily.

**Figure 4.22** Quadruped single arm raise. This exercise, together with those shown in Figures 4.23 and 4.24, helps to condition the muscles of the entire back. This is particularly important in patients susceptible to osteoporosis, because the pull of these muscles on the skeleton helps maintain bone calcium. This exercise looks easy, but it can also easily increase back pain. It should not be attempted until back pain has been infrequent and minimal in intensity for at least 1 month.

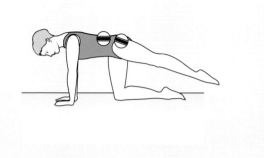

**Figure 4.23** Quadruped single leg raise. The aim of this exercise is to strengthen the buttock, posterior thigh, and lower back muscles in a back-protected position. Hold your chin in. Look down at the floor. Do a pelvic pinch and raise your left leg about 8–10 cm (3–4 inches) off the floor. Avoid extension of your back. Hold the raised leg and count from 1001 to 1006. Put your leg down and relax. *Do not allow your back to sway.* Repeat the exercise, raising your right leg as instructed. See Figure 4.22 for sequence repetitions.

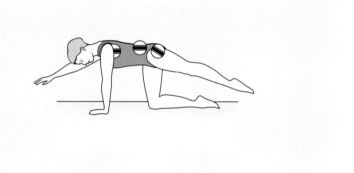

**Figure 4.24** Quadruped contralateral arm and leg raise. The aim of this exercise is to simultaneously strengthen the muscles on each side of the spine, to improve coordination and control. Hold your chin in. Look down at the floor. Do a pelvic pinch and raise your left leg about 8–10 cm (3–4 inches) off the floor. Raise your right arm about 30 cm (1 foot) off the floor. Hold and count from 1001 to 1006. Relax *without swaying your back.* Repeat the exercise, raising your right leg and your left arm as instructed above. See Figure 4.22 for sequence repetitions. *Caution:* Stop the exercise if back or leg pain increases.

101

TABLE 4.6

**Maintenance exercises\* for patients with mild low back pain, to be done once daily**

| Exercise | Repetitions/holds |
| --- | --- |
| **Sedentary person** | |
| Pelvic tilt | 3 |
| Single knee to chest | 3 |
| Partial sit-up or knee push with chair | Up to 40 seconds |
| Double knee to chest | 3 |
| Supine hamstring stretch | 2 |
| Beginning pelvic rotation | 3 |
| Wall slide 30° angle | Up to 40 seconds |
| Supine single straight leg raise | 5 |
| **Active person** | |
| Pelvic tilt | 2 |
| Double knee to chest | 3 |
| Supine hamstring stretch | 2 |
| Partial sit-up | 40 seconds |
| Crossed hip rotator stretch | 2 |
| Advanced pelvic rotation | 3 |
| Supine hamstring stretch (opposite leg) | 2 |
| Quadruped contralateral arm and leg raise | 40 seconds |
| Calf stretch (standing) | 1 each side |
| Wall slide repetitions | 20 |
| Back bends (standing) | 5 |

\*See the list on page 8 to find each exercise

**Conservative management – Key points**

- Pain management during the acute first 4-week phase of low back pain should consist of RICE (rest, ice, corset/brace, exercise) unless 'red flags' are present. No x-ray or laboratory investigation is indicated unless 'red flags' are present.
- Treatment will depend on assessment of severity (severe, moderate, mild, minimal). Multidisciplinary treatment should be strongly considered in chronic pain management.
- Medications during the acute phase can include acetaminophen (paracetamol), NSAIDs and possibly muscle relaxants. Short-term opioids for severe pain can also be considered.
- The VAS (visual analog scale) for measuring pain is very helpful.
- Bed rest is rarely indicated, but restful postures and ergonomic considerations to promote comfortable ambulatory activities should be encouraged.
- Graduated and progressive home reconditioning along with pain control measures are indicated.
- Spinal manipulation once or twice weekly for up to 4 weeks may be helpful.
- Acupuncture may be helpful. A trial of six to eight treatments should help determine acupuncture efficacy.
- Corsets are of equivocal benefit for acute pain management.

**Key reference**

Le Doux MS, Langford KH. Spinal cord stimulation for failed back syndrome. *Spine* 1993;18:191–4.

Herkowitz HN, Garfin SR, Balderston RA et al., eds. *Rothman–Simeone: The Spine*, 4th edn. Philadelphia: *WB Saunders*, 1999.

Mayer TG, Mooney V, Gatchel RJ. *Contemporary Conservative Care for Painful Spinal Disorders*. Philadelphia: Lee & Febiger, 1991.

Nachemson AL, Jonsson E. *Neck and Back Pain: the Scientific Evidence of Causes, Diagnosis and Treatment*. Baltimore: Lippincott, Williams & Wilkins, 2000.

Swezey RL, ed. Low back pain. *Phys Med Rehabil Clin N Am* 1998;9:309–523.

Swezey RL, Swezey AM. *Good News For Bad Backs*. Santa Monica, California: Cequal, 2002.

## Injection therapies

When/if the various conservative measures have proved ineffective, too slow in providing adequate relief or poorly tolerated, injection options can be considered. For refractory areas of focal pain, i.e. trigger points or tender points (see page 43), injection of a local anesthetic (e.g. 3–5 mL of 2% lidocaine without epinephrine/adrenaline) into a tender muscle trigger point can give relief. A small amount of corticosteroid, e.g. 3–10 mg of triamcinolone or betamethasone, can be added for anti-inflammatory therapy to the area of the tender point at a tendon or ligamentous enthesis.

**Epidural injections** are mainly used to relieve refractory sciatic nerve root pain, dysesthesias and/or associated paresis. They are also used to relieve symptoms of neurogenic claudication associated with lumbar spinal stenosis. Epidural injections may help induce or expedite a remission of symptoms and so avoid a surgical intervention. They can also provide periods of significant symptom relief when other treatments have failed, and for those patients who are high-risk and therefore not candidates for surgery.

Epidural injections are not without risk, however. It has been reported that as many as 30% of epidural injections administered by experienced clinicians without fluoroscopic monitoring are not properly placed in the epidural space, and this not only nullifies any benefit, but adds the potential risks of an inadvertent spinal tap (headache, infection, hemorrhage and cost) to the known risks of moderate-to-high doses of corticosteroids. Epidural injections should always be expertly administered under fluoroscopic visualization, so that the possibility of a therapeutic response is high and the likelihood of inadvertent needle placement is minimized.

The duration of full or partial remission following an epidural corticosteroid injection may be days to a few months. In the case of acute radiculopathy, this may be sufficient to permit nerve root and discal inflammation to subside sufficiently for healing to occur. In the case of spinal stenosis with associated neurogenic claudication, an epidural injection every few months may permit more comfortable walking and standing, an improved quality of life, and postpone or possibly rule out surgical interventions.

**Nerve root canal injections** are performed under fluoroscopic visualization to enhance precision and minimize the risk of inadvertent needle placement. They are indicated for refractory nerve root impingement syndromes where conservative measures have proved inadequate, and where clinical, radiographic and electrodiagnostic procedures can, with reasonable precision, identify the locus of the root canal neural compression.

Nerve root canal injections performed under fluoroscopic guidance carry similar risks to those associated with epidural injections. Although the corticosteroid dose is usually lower, the risk of trauma in a tight nerve root canal is greater.

There is no guarantee that symptoms will be relieved by a nerve root canal injection, or that, even if properly performed, the intervention will relieve pain or restore useful function to weakened muscles.

**Facet (zygapophyseal) joint injection.** Fluoroscopic guidance now allows precise needle placement into the facet joint for therapeutic injections. In an early study, injections of 3 mL of 5% hypertonic saline into facet joints provoked immediate local deep, dull pain in both symptomatic patients and asymptomatic controls. After 20 seconds the pain spread in a sclerotomal distribution to the buttocks and posterior thigh and trochanteric region. It was then relieved by an intra-articular injection of a local anesthetic. Subsequent studies, however, have not produced consistent results with regard to relief of symptoms, arthrographic findings, or responses to intra-articular anesthetic injections. Patients over age 65 whose low back pain was not aggravated by coughing, hyperextension, flexion or arising from flexion, or extension-rotation, and was relieved by recumbency, were the most likely to respond.

*Facet joint denervation.* Because of the overlapping enervation between facet joints, stimulating and/or relieving the pain in one joint is non-specific and cannot identify the source of the back pain. Various facet joint neural denervations have been attempted, using freezing and thermal radio-frequency irradiation, as well as local phenol injections and rhizotomy. None of these methods, however, has proved superior to the others, nor are any currently widely used (because of the lack of consistent responses).

*Facet joint corticosteroid injections* share many of the above uncertainties because of the ambiguity of the symptoms and the poor correlation between symptoms and demonstrable facet joint pathology. Typically, both the L4–L5 and L5–S1 facet joints on the symptomatic side are injected with a corticosteroid, because of the difficulty in determining the symptomatic facet joint and because, with the exception of post-traumatic or scoliosis-related disorders, the lower facet joints (like the lower disks) are most often pathologically and presumably clinically involved.

*Facet joint synovial cyst corticosteroid injection.* Facet joint synovial cysts are not uncommonly found on MRI studies for low back and sciatic pain disorders. They may contribute to the symptomatology, and recede after percutaneous, image-guided intrasynovial facet joint corticosteroid injections.

**Sacroiliac joint injection.** Despite the ambiguities in the clinical assessment of sacroiliac dysfunctions, almost all patients with suspected non-inflammatory sacroiliac joint pain recover spontaneously or with conservative therapies. For those few who do not improve, sacroiliac corticosteroid joint injections can be performed under fluoroscopic guidance in a manner similar to that used for facet joint injection. In one study, the sacroiliac joint was injected with lidocaine after visualization of the joint with contrast medium. Those patients who showed a positive response in terms of pain reduction on moving the sacroiliac joint area then received injections of betamethasone and lidocaine. Physical therapy was continued, and if improvement was not sustained, a second injection was given. Although far from conclusive, this suggests that sacroiliac joint pain may be responsive to intra-articular corticosteroid injections.

**Intrabursal injection.** Regardless of the precise pathogenesis, local corticosteroid injections into tender bursas can often provide prompt pain relief. Large doses of corticosteroids are not required, as these bursas respond to injections of as little as 5 mg of triamcinolone, or its equivalent, in 2–5 mL of 1% lidocaine.

## Surgery

Low back pain, with or without sciatica, generally improves over time. Surgery, in contrast, is far from uniformly successful and carries a burden of operative and postoperative mortality and morbidity. Despite this, surgery is necessary in some cases, and particularly in some of the patients with a 'red flag' (see Table 2.1 on page 33). To delay urgently-indicated surgery for loss of bowel and bladder control in acute cauda equina syndromes, or for major loss of muscular control not responsive to conservative measures including nerve root and/or epidural cortico-steroid injections, risks potentially far greater damage. The decision to operate, and if so when, is dependent on the severity of the discomfort and the potential for functional impairment that might be avoided by a surgical procedure. Before that point is reached, both the physician and the patient must agree that all reasonable conservative measures have been considered and, when feasible, given an adequate trial.

Expectations that a properly performed and appropriate operation will expedite the relief of pain and discomfort are usually realistic, but outcome perceptions depend on the type of questions asked, and at what point in the postoperative period they are asked. Satisfactory outcomes have ranged from 60% to 97%, depending on questionnaire design. Good results from appropriate surgery by expert surgeons have been reported to give complete relief of leg pain in 73% of patients and complete relief of back pain in 63%. Unfortunately, some patients with initially good outcomes regress, though a few with poor outcomes also improve.

After careful analysis, the Cochrane Review concluded that: 'There is considerable evidence on the clinical effectiveness of discectomy for carefully selected patients with sciatica caused by lumbar disk prolapse that fails to resolve with conservative management. There is no scientific evidence on the effectiveness of any form of surgical decompression or fusion for degenerative lumbar spondylosis compared with natural history, placebo, or conservative management.'

**Open microdiscectomy** is now the procedure of choice for disk herniations, both contained and non-contained. The procedure consists of inserting a magnifying loupe or microscope through a small laminotomy to guide removal of the protruded or extruded disk material. A major concern is that the nerve root is not adequately exposed and may be traumatized during the discectomy. Most patients with symptoms of nerve root compression respond, but 7% may experience a recurrence. Patients can usually go almost straight back to work, and the mean time for return to work is 1.5 weeks.

Microdiscectomy for back pain, as opposed to radiculopathy, is less successful. The most common complication is a missed pathological disk or discal fragment because of the limited visual exposure and the lack of precision of the diagnostic methods. As in all spinal surgery, there is a risk of infection, dural tears, hemorrhage and postoperative arachnoidal scarring.

**Percutaneous surgical discectomy** procedures are minimally invasive, but have not yet proved to be reliably effective, and their futures remain in doubt. Their efficacy is significantly limited by the restricted view of any extruded disk material. These procedures use surgical approaches to shrink the nucleus and relieve its painful pressures, in a similar way to percutaneous chymopapain nucleolysis, which used an enzymic approach. The chymopapain procedure was associated with complications and was far from predictably more effective than conservative treatment, however, and it is now seldom used.

*Percutaneous suction discectomy* uses a rotary cutting device that is inserted into the nucleus percutaneously. The results are no better than with the chymopapain procedure, and the costs are higher than for microdiscectomy.

*Percutaneous laser discectomy* uses laser energy to perform the discectomy. The results have not lived up to expectation, and this expensive procedure carries the additional risk of thermal damage to the vertebral end-plate and neural tissues.

*Percutaneous thermal intradiscal catheters* have been tried in a small series of patients with low back pain who would otherwise have been treated with a lumbar fusion procedure. A measure of pain relief was obtained by about 75% of the 25 patients after 7 months.

**Artificial disk replacements** consist of a polyethylene core between two metal plates, designed to replace a dysfunctional disk and permit partial (50–60%) restoration of intervertebral movement. The procedure involves an anterior, intra-abdominal approach and 2 days of hospitalization. Their longer term efficacy remains to be established.

**Lumbar fusion** is usually performed by one of three different techniques:
• anterior interbody fusion
• posterior fusion
• intertransverse process fusion.
The last of these appears to give the best overall success rate. Anterior discectomies with and without fusion have not proved as successful as laminotomy and disk fragment excision and are now seldom performed.

In addition to radiographic evidence of lumbar instability and low back pain, regardless of the cause, lumbar fusions are performed to permit spinal stabilization for extensive foraminotomies with facetectomies for neural decompressions and to stabilize a symptomatic pseudoarthrosis. Disk herniation with spondylolisthesis typically occurs at the level above the slippage, and only very occasionally at the same level, in which case a fusion of the spondylolisthesis is usually performed.

There is on average a 10–15% non-union rate for single-level, instrument-stabilized fusions, and this increases to 30–40% for three-level fusions. With predominant slippage at L4–L5, failure to fuse the L5–S1 resulted in only a 55% success rate for the surgical fusion. Even in surgically successful lumbar fusions, only about one-third of patients with L4–S1 degenerative spondylosis and chronic low back pain unresponsive to previous conservative therapies obtain some measure of pain relief, because the association of the mechanical and degenerative abnormalities and the pain is often not clear. Lumbar fusions are associated with significant complications, with an overall complication rate of 17% in one large series (related primarily to pedicle screw fixation), and with twice the mortality rate of non-fusion options.

*New approaches.* Posterior and anterior fusions have been tried with different types of bone implants, and with metal and non-metal pedicle-screw-attached semi-flexible devices, in an attempt to shorten the operating time and trauma while lengthening the durability of the intervertebral fusion. The latest techniques using instillation of bone morphogenic proteins to stimulate intradiscal bony fusion appear promising. Recent trials of the use of metallic-threaded fusion cages installed endoscopically have reported radiographic fusion in 96% of cases and clinical improvement in 89%, without significant complications.

*Vertebroplasty and kyphoplasty* are the newest methods for stabilizing a lumbar fracture. In both methods, a poly(methyl methacrylate) (PMMA) bone cement is instilled into the vertebral fracture site. In kyphoplasty, two inflatable bone tamps are inserted percutaneously into the affected vertebra and then inflated to raise the vertebral end-plate and at least partly restore the bone height lost by the compression fracture.

Vertebroplasty and kyphoplasty are used primarily to treat osteoporotic fractures, but they are also used to treat painful primary or metastatic vertebral tumors. Vertebroplasty is reported to produce pain relief in 70–90% of cases, and early results indicate pain relief in 90% at 18 months for kyphoplasty. Both procedures utilize a percutaneous needle to guide the injection of PMMA and can be performed on an outpatient basis, and provide prompt and sustainable relief of the compression fracture pain. Vertebroplasty antedates kyphoplasty and was first utilized in 1984 in France and in the USA in 1994, and therefore has had a wider utilization and a greater long-term experience. Kyphoplasty, in addition to restoring some (about 50%) of the lost vertebral height and thereby improving posture and cardiorespiratory function, has the added advantage of containing the bone cement within the tamps for the time (about 1 hour) that it takes to harden, which reduces the risk of cement leakage into the spinal canal. These procedures have so far proved safe and maintained fracture stabilization.

---

**Injections and surgery – Key points**

- Epidural and/or nerve root canal injections are safer and more reliable if done with fluoroscopic monitoring.
- Intrabursal and tender-point injections with low-dose steroids can often provide prompt pain reduction.
- Surgery is usually effective for refractory sciatica but is of equivocal benefit for low back pain. Approximately one-third of successful spine fusions provide pain relief for chronic low back pain.
- Vertebroplasties and kyphoplasties can provide prompt pain control in osteoporotic or malignant vertebral fractures.

---

**Key references**

Barendse GAM, van den Berg SGM, Kessels AHF et al. Randomized controlled trial of percutaneous intradiscal radiofrequency thermocoagulation for chronic discogenic back pain: lack of effect from a 90-second 70°C lesion. *Spine* 2001;26:287–92.

Facisczewski T, McKiernan F. Calling all vertebral fractures: classification of vertebral compression fractures: a consensus for comparison of treatment and outcome. *J Bone Miner Res* 2002;17:185–91.

Fritzell P, Hagg O, Wessberg P, Nordwall A, Swedish Lumbar Spine Study Group. 2001 Volvo Award Winner in clinical studies: lumbar fusion versus nonsurgical treatment for chronic low back pain. *Spine* 2001;26:2521–34.

Garfin SR, Hansen AY, Reiley MA. New technologies in spine: kyphoplasty and vertebroplasty for the treatment of painful osteoporotic compression fractures. *Spine* 2001; 26:1511–15.

Kaplan M, Dreyfuss P, Halbrook B, Bogduk N. The ability of lumbar medial branch blocks to anesthetize the zygapophyseal joint. *Spine* 1998;23:1847–52.

Revel M, Poiraudeau S, Auleley G et al. Capacity of the clinical picture to characterize low back pain relieved by facet joint anesthesia. Proposed criteria to identify patients with painful facet joints. *Spine* 1998;23:1972–6.

Saal JA, Saal JS. Intradiscal electrothermal treatment for chronic discogenic low back pain: prospective outcome study with a minimum 2-year follow-up. *Spine* 2002;27: 966–74.

Schwarzer AC, Derby R, Aprill CN et al. The value of the provocation response in lumbar zygapophyseal joint injections. *Clin J Pain* 2000; 10:309–13.

Swezey RL, ed. Low back pain. *Phys Med Rehabil Clin N Am* 1998;9:309–523.

Low back pain is an almost inevitable fact of life. It can range from an acute, severely painful episode, to a chronic disabling condition with profound individual and social consequences. Physicians can anticipate that this millennium will continue to challenge them, and their patients, with back pain problems and with the rapidly growing number of diagnostic and therapeutic options from which to choose.

The good news is that most patients will recover, either spontaneously or with some measure of help from a physician. The less welcome news is that despite the amazing array of sophisticated diagnostic methods, it is still very difficult to identify the exact basis for an individual's back pain, and this leads in turn to very difficult choices. Should nothing be done, because all testing has too great a share of false positives? Or given society's increasing recourse to litigation, should all possible diagnostic tools be used to avoid any possibility of a missed diagnosis? If the 'red flags' are up, there may be no choice but to aggressively pursue any potentially life-threatening or crippling possibility.

The same disturbing choices are faced when it comes to treatment. As most patients with low back pain recover spontaneously, and as any treatment may produce an untoward side-effect, perhaps nothing is better than something. If this approach is taken, however, many patients will do something for themselves, which may be less than therapeutic. The physician must choose wisely and well, provide support and guidance to patients, and 'comfort always'.

This program is designed to gradually warm the muscles so that they can be more easily stretched. The exercises are performed in the morning before breakfast, and can also be used to warm up and cool down before and after athletic activity. The warm-up exercises are performed with each leg in turn and repeated five times at increasing tempo. The strengthening and conditioning exercises are also repeated on each side where appropriate.

**Loosening-up stretches**

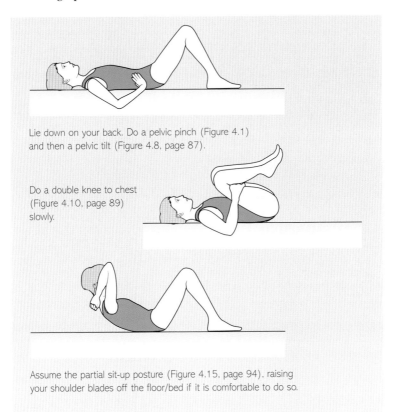

Lie down on your back. Do a pelvic pinch (Figure 4.1) and then a pelvic tilt (Figure 4.8, page 87).

Do a double knee to chest (Figure 4.10, page 89) slowly.

Assume the partial sit-up posture (Figure 4.15, page 94), raising your shoulder blades off the floor/bed if it is comfortable to do so.

## The rhythm and pacing warm-up

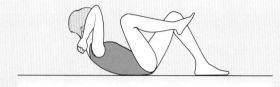

Move 1: First, bring one knee to your chest.

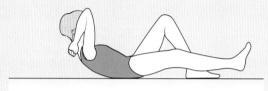

Move 2: Keeping the right heel just off the floor/bed, straighten the right leg fully so that the leg is just off the floor/bed. This is the starting position.

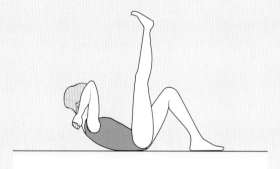

Move 3: Vertical leg raise, keeping the leg straight.

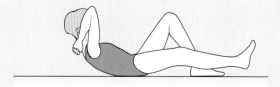

Move 4: Return to the starting position.

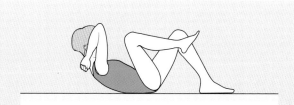

Move 5: Knee to chest.

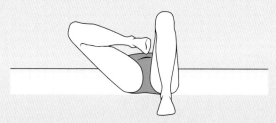

Move 6: Rotate your bent leg outward into a frog-leg position. Keep the knee and leg as horizontal as possible while straightening the leg.

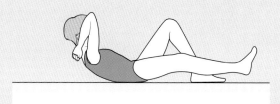

Turn the foot up vertically when you are again at the starting position.

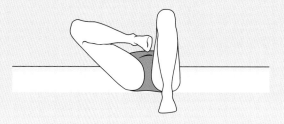

Move 7: Return the knee to the chest, keeping the knee in the frog-leg position and in the horizontal plane.

117

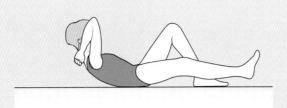

Move 8: Straighten the leg, keeping it just off the floor/bed, and return to the starting position.

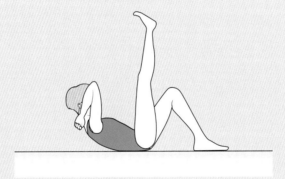

Move 9: Repeat the vertical leg raise.

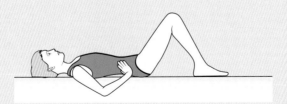

Move 10: Bend the knee and place the foot back on the floor/bed. Repeat the entire series with the opposite leg.

## Strengthening and conditioning exercises

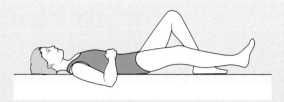

Hold a 6-second single straight leg raise (Figure 4.12) on each side with as much effort as you can possibly make.

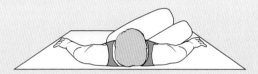

Do a beginning pelvic rotation (Figure 4.14) slowly to each side. If comfortable, do two to three more slowly on each side.

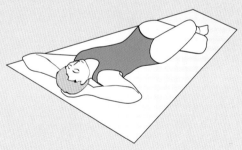

Do an advanced pelvic rotation (Figure 4.18) slowly to each side. If comfortable, do another to the right and hold for a count of 1001, 1002.

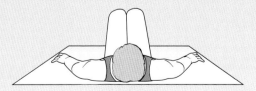

Return to the basic pelvic tilt position and lower your head and shoulders to the floor. Repeat the advanced pelvic rotation on the left side.

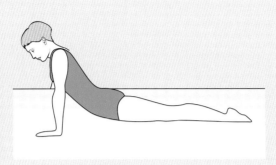

Roll over onto your abdomen and do five press-ups, keeping your pelvis on the bed/floor.

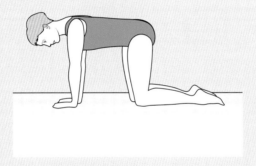

Assume the quadruped position.

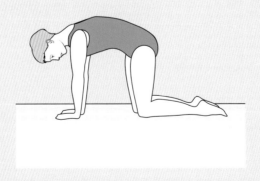

Arch your back and hold a cat-back posture (Figure 4.21, page 99).

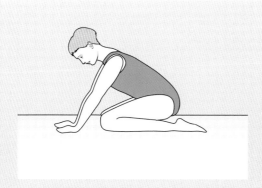

The sit-back stretch. Keeping your hands in place, sit back on your heels.

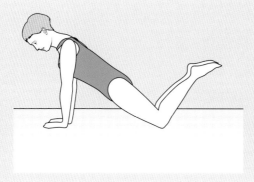

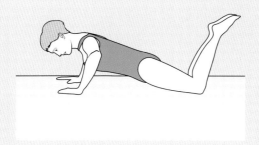

The partial push-up. Do a push-up with knees bent (or, if you can without arching your back, a full push-up) and hold, with your elbows bent, for a count of 10–25. Alternatively, do 5–20 slow push-ups (knees bent or knees straight) under full back-stabilized control.

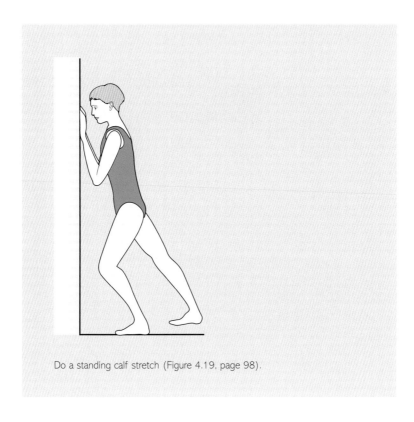

Do a standing calf stretch (Figure 4.19, page 98).

# Sources of further information

## USA

American Academy of Physical
Medicine & Rehabilitation
One IBM Plaza, Suite 2500
Chicago, IL 60611-3604
Tel: 312 464 9700
Fax: 312 464 0227
info@aapmr.org
www.aapmr.org

American College of Rheumatology
1800 Century Place, Suite 250
Atlanta, GA 30345-4300
Tel: 404 633 3777
Fax: 404 633 1870
acr@rheumatology.org
www.rheumatology.org

American Occupational Therapy
Association
PO Box 31220
Bethesda, MD 20824-1220
www.aota.org

American Physical Therapy
Association
1111 North Fairfax Street
Alexandria, VA 22314-1488
Tel: 1 800 999 2782 (toll free) or
703 684 2782
Fax: 703 684 7343
www.apta.org

The National Fibromyalgia
Partnership
140 Zinn Way
Linden, VA 22642-5609
Tel: 1 866 725 4404 (toll free)
Fax: 540 622 2988
www.fmpartnership.org

National Arthritis Foundation
PO Box 7669
Atlanta, GA 30357-0669
Tel: 1 800 283 7800
Research-funding enquiries:
Research Department
Arthritis Foundation
1330 West Peachtree St
Atlanta, GA 30309
Tel: 404 965 7537
www.arthritis.org

National Institute of Arthritis and
Musculoskeletal and Skin Diseases
National Institutes of Health
1 AMS Circle
Bethesda, MD 20892-3675
www.niams.nih.gov

National Osteoporosis Foundation
1232 22nd Street NW
Washington, DC 20037-1292
Tel: 202 223 2226
www.nof.org

North American Spine Society
22 Calendar Court, 2nd Floor
LaGrange, IL 60525
Tel: 877 774 6337 (toll free)
info@spine.org
www.spine.org

Spondylitis Association of America
14827 Ventura Blvd, #222
Sherman Oaks, CA 91403
Tel: 800 777 8189 (toll free); 818
981 1616
info@spondylitis.org
www.spondylitis.org

Scleroderma Foundation
12 Kent Way, Suite 101
Byfield, MA 01922
Tel: 800 722 4673 (toll free); 978
463 5843
Fax: 978 463 5809
sfinfo@scleroderma.org
www.scleroderma.org

Yoga.com
87 Freshpond Parkway
Cambridge, MA 01238
USA
Tel: 1 866 266 9642 (toll free)
Fax: 253 679 2195
staff@yoga.com
www.yoga.com

Yoga Research and Education
Center
2400A County Center Drive
Santa Rosa, CA 95403
USA
Tel: 707 566 9000
mail@yrec.org
www.yrec.org/

Yoga Journal
2054 University Avenue
Berkeley
CA 94704
USA
Tel: 510 841 9200
Fax: 510 644 3101
www.yogajournal.com

The Pilates Method Alliance
PO Box 370906
Miami, FL 33137-0906
USA
Tel: 1 866 573 4945 (toll free)
info@pilatesmethodalliance.org
www.pilatesmethodalliance.org/

Stott Pilates
Suite 1402
2200 Yonge Street
Toronto, Ontario M4S 2C6
Canada
Tel (North America): 1 800 910
0001 (toll free) or 416 482 4050
Tel (UK): 0800 328 5676
Fax: 416 482 2742
www.stottpilates.com

Local Guide – Pilates
www.aolsvc.digitalcity.com/
pilatesclasses/

Rolf Institute for Structural
Integration
205 Canyon Boulevard
Boulder, CO 80302
USA
Tel: 800 530 8875
Fax: 303 449 5978
www.rolf.org/

Academy of Mensendieck
Specialists
PO Box 19450
Stanford, CA 94309-9450
USA
Tel: 650 8518184
Fax: 650 8513742
www.backfitness.com

## UK/Europe
BackCare
(charity registered as The
National Back Pain Association)
16 Elmtree Road
Teddington
Middlesex, TW11 8ST
Tel: 020 8977 5474
Fax: 020 8943 5318
www.backpain.org

British Chiropractic Association
Blagrave House
17 Blagrave Street
Reading, Berkshire, RG1 1QB
Tel: 0118 950 5950
Fax: 0118 958 8946
enquiries@chiropractic-uk.co.uk
www.chiropractic-uk.co.uk

British Osteopathic Association
boa@osteopathy.org
www.osteopathy.org

British Society for Rheumatology
41 Eagle Street
London WC1R 4TL
Tel: 0207 242 3313
Fax: 0207 242 3277
bsr@rheumatology.org.uk
www.rheumatology.org.uk

Chartered Society of Physiotherapy
14 Bedford Row
London WC1R 4ED
Tel: 020 7306 6666
Fax: 020 7306 6611
www.csp.org.uk

The Society for Back Pain Research
The British Orthopaedic
Association
35–43 Lincoln's Inn Fields
London WC1A 3PN

Pilates Foundation UK Limited
PO Box 36052
London, SW16 1XQ
UK
Tel: 07071 781 859
Fax: 020 8696 0088
admin@pilates.foundation
www.pilatesfoundation.com

Body Control Pilates Association
6 Langley Street
London
WC2H 9JA
Tel: 020 7379 3734
Fax: 020 7379 7551
info@bodycontrol.co.uk
www.bodycontrol.co.uk/

European Rolfing Association
Kapuzinerstrasse 25
80337 München
Germany
Tel: + 49 89 543 709 40
www.rolfing.org/

**Other websites**
The Yoga Site
www.yogasite.com

Yogafinder.com
www.yogafinder.com/

International Sivananda Yoga
Vedanta Centers
www.sivananda.org/

Aussie Pilates
www.pilates.net/

# Index

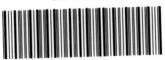